Balancing Diabetes

Conversations about finding happiness and living well

Kerri Sparling

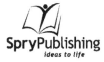

SpryPublishing
ideas to life

This edition is published by Spry Publishing LLC
315 East Eisenhower Pkwy, Ste 2
Ann Arbor, MI 48108 USA

Printed and bound in the United States of America.

10 9 8 7 6 5 4 3 2

Library of Congress Control Number: 2013949026

Paperback ISBN: 978-1-938170-37-9
E-book ISBN: 978-1-938170-38-6

for my littlest bird

Contents

Chapter One

Making Sense of the New Normal

When I was two years old, I tripped and fell, smashing my nose against the stone hearth that surrounded our fireplace. The blood! My little face! My parents freaking out! There were exclamation points everywhere, and, to this day, my nose still has a bit of a bump to it where the cartilage hit the stone.

I was so little that the memory is lost forever to me, but my parents remember it distinctly. Like so much of my early childhood—the only years I have had without type 1 diabetes—these memories are caught in snapshots and half-fictionalized stories we repeat around the dinner table at holidays.

However, I do remember wetting the bed before my diagnosis. I was six years old and frustrated by my perceived lack of self-control. "Mom, I can't stop!" was my lament, and she shared my frustration because she couldn't help me stop. I have a very clear memory of walking downstairs to the living room where my parents were watching television and throwing my "lovey blanket" into the middle of the floor.

"I can't stop peeing in my bed! But I can stop sucking my thumb," I said, jutting my chin out and making what has evolved into my "stubborn fool" face. "I'm DONE." (My parents remind me of this story every time I get my mind set on doing something new and frustratingly challenging. *"You always do what you can do, and what you can't control, you still try to control,"* they say. I'm still not sure if this is a compliment.)

After the purchase of a system, worn in my underpants, that detected the presence of urine by announcing it with an alarm that pierced through the quiet night of our home and vaulted me from my bed, the nighttime accidents stopped almost entirely. But I was still up once or twice a night using the bathroom.

It was months later, during a before-school physical that included the standard pee-in-the-cup moment that our pediatrician, Dr. L, came out with a urine sample in his hand. "Whose pee is this?" he asked, pointing to the cup with the bright blue lid.

"That's Kerri's," my mom said, assigning the sample as mine and not my brother's.

"It's a little high in sugar. She needs to go to the hospital for blood work this afternoon," he indicated.

According to my mom, who remembers this day clearly while my memory is cluttered more with the clowns on the bathroom wallpaper in the office, there wasn't much explanation about the test or what it was for. The blood draw for a seven year old felt more acute and more dramatic than the vague "high in sugar" diagnosis it was confirming.

But then came the phone call and a conversation between my mom and the doctor. He told her that my blood sugar was 250 mg/dL and that I had "juvenile diabetes." In a controlled panic, my mother was calling my father and saying that word again—diabetes—and making arrangements to take me to Rhode Island Hospital the next day.

When I talked about my diagnosis with my mother over cups of tea years later, I asked her about how she felt upon receiving that call and being handed my diagnosis. She shared, "*I wasn't scared. I wasn't panicked. I knew that [our extended family friend] Eleanor's son, Jim, had diabetes, but I didn't know what that meant or what it entailed. It wasn't me being tough, but more that I didn't know what we were getting in to. I just thought, 'Okay, let's go deal with this, whatever this is.'*"

She continued, "*We were sent home with a urine testing kit—do you remember those test tubes and the little color-changing tabs we'd drop in?*"

I did remember those. The test tubes would turn orange and get hot if my blood sugar was too high.

"*When the tubes stayed cool and the color was closer to*

blue, it meant 'good job!' and that your urine didn't contain too much sugar. The thing is, home glucose meters existed when you were diagnosed, but we weren't given one. And, for the first month, I was okay with the urine tests, because that's all I could handle at the time. It was so much to take in and so much to learn that adding in all the numbers was more than I could adjust to.

"We eventually got a meter when we went to Joslin Diabetes Center for the first time about five weeks after you were diagnosed. For that first month, I had been adjusting to the needles and the insulin and the sliding scale of insulin doses, but I was starting to get frustrated at the imperfect science of urine testing. I was ready for more information, and that's when we went to Boston to see a pediatric endocrinologist."

When pressed to recall memories of my diagnosis, I have a hard time coming up with much. Most of my young life was a flurry of events and memories that I don't remember diabetes being a part of, even though I know it was there the whole time. Growing up, I didn't have a "diabetes community" to speak of, and for many years, my family and I dealt with diabetes on our own.

When my then-boyfriend/now-husband and I started dating, I mentioned to him that I didn't know anyone else who was living with diabetes. I had found plenty of people who died from it and grim accounts as to how and why by searching online, though.

"Have you ever considered blogging?" he asked, innocently. That very question is how I ended up sharing personal details about my chronic illness and its emotional and physical influence on my life on the Internet for the world to read.

In May of 2005, at the encouragement of my boyfriend, I started a blog in hopes of connecting with other adults who were living with type 1 diabetes and who were actually *living*. I knew there were complications that could arise as a result of this disease and I knew the day-to-day was challenging in its own way, but I was in search of people who were doing normal things—dating, going on job interviews, having fun—with type 1 diabetes as just part of the bigger equation.

A diabetes diagnosis is only the first of so many "new normals." As a kid, my parents and I both needed to learn how to pinch hit for my busted pancreas, making sense of the new tools and new medications introduced into my young life. The point of all that excellent care and attention was to help me grow up and become an adult with a life of my own. Which, eerily enough, actually *happened*.

Now that I am an adult, I find a new version of "normal" to adjust to every few years. At first, I went to college and needed to find balance in being almost solely responsible for my own care, making sure my medical needs were met without my parents looking over my shoulder. Then, it became the "new normal" of life in my own apartment, without roommates, balancing blood sugar checks against nights out with my friends and keeping up with the constantly shifting sands of medical insurance and a "real job." Now, as an adult with a family, I'm trying to figure out how to keep my health afloat in the flow of life as a writer, a wife, and the mother of a little girl.

For the first few weeks as I dove into the world of blogging and started actively sharing my health and my emotional ties to diabetes with the Internet, I thought my needs were unique. I thought I might be the only person with diabetes (PWD) who was struggling to make sense of this disease, but I was also gripped by this strange, unrelenting hunger to connect with a community that understood, intrinsically, what I was going through each day.

"Do other diabetics think about this stuff?" I asked out loud to my boyfriend. He shrugged his shoulders, unsure. "Am I a weirdo for wanting to find other people who don't make their own insulin?"

Then something life-changing happened ... I discovered my peer group online. I saw that I wasn't the exception. Especially in the space where people were actively disclosing their diabetes in discussion forums and blogs, I saw that I was the norm. You see, diabetes, even when classified as "no big deal," plays a role in shaping who we are and who we become. As a disease, it doesn't get to take credit for our successes, but it may be a driving force in getting us there.

Scott Johnson was one of the first writers I found online who was writing about a real life with diabetes. Similar to me, he didn't remember much about his diagnosis and he was looking to share his story in hopes of finding others like him. *"I was only five years old when I was diagnosed, so every memory about that time is very vague. I remember watching an old war movie on TV, and the nurse coming in to give me Nilla Wafers as a snack. But that's kind of it.*

But as I grew up, I realized it was hard to live with diabetes. And for those who ask if it makes a difference because I don't remember a 'before,' I can say that I'm aware of what life would be like without diabetes. I see all these other people not doing what I'm required to do. I see the extra stuff. But it makes me feel strong because I feel like I'm kicking butt at life most of the time, and I'm doing it all with diabetes. Knowing that made me want to share my story, to prove that this can be done."

What makes this happen? Instinctively, you'd think there isn't a shred of balance to be found in focusing anything at all on a disease. Shouldn't a person living with a chronic illness ignore it at all costs, save for the necessary medical management required to stay alive? Doesn't focusing on it too much make it overwhelming—a dominating factor? What grace and balance can be achieved from bringing diabetes into the "other" parts of your life—your hobbies, your job, or even the friendships you forge?

You'd be surprised. I am constantly surprised.

Clearly, not everyone wants to have diabetes bleed out (terrible pun, but I'm going with it) into other aspects of their lives, and I have tremendous respect for people who achieve great things that have nothing to do with diabetes. But I do have a special level of respect and appreciation for people who take this disease and make it a bigger part of their life, as a way of achieving peace, understanding, and, hopefully, balance. There are so many examples of people who have immersed themselves in the diabetes community, both in an offline sense and through the magic of the Internet, and give back in a way that helps others find that same peace, understanding, and balance.

Ryan Noonan was probably the first other kid with diabetes I ever encountered because we went to the same school system and his older brother was in my class. Diagnosed at the age of nine, Ryan struggled to find balance with diabetes for much of his life, dealing with his disease by ignoring it as much as he could while growing up. *"It is very easy to say but a lot tougher to do—don't worry about what other people think. I worried about what everyone thought or said for far too long and it did a lot of damage to me as a person, but mostly as a diabetic. I was so worried about making everyone else happy that I wasn't happy myself. Do your own thing—you know what is right and what is wrong. Diabetes has made me a much stronger person, a person who will take control of a situation if needed. And work-wise, I've had the confidence to set up meetings with people I wouldn't have had the guts to say hi to in person before.*

But the biggest step I had to take is one toward taking total responsibility for my diabetes. In the past, I would say

I couldn't eat something or participate in a certain activity because I had diabetes. I found that as my diabetes control improved, I felt like I could do more, in every aspect of my life. If, and when, you need help on your way, please trust me that you need to ask for that help. But at the end of the day, if your blood sugar is in-range, then you're doing something right."

When it comes to diabetes management, "doing the right thing" covers a whole slate of actions and emotions. An elevated level of responsibility seems to come in tandem with the diagnosis of diabetes when you're young. I felt this myself, being handed my mortality at such a young age. "Hey, you know this can kill you, right? So take care of yourself" was something that doctors and relatives alike would say to me, making me acutely aware of how fragile life can be. While many of my friends went through a period of invincibility, I never hit stride with that mentality. Instead, I had a heightened awareness of how vulnerable my health was and I worked hard to maintain the health baseline that seemed to come so naturally for my friends who didn't have health concerns.

I met Abby Bayer through my childhood diabetes camp, Clara Barton Camp (affectionately known as CBC). The entire camp was designed so that all campers, staffers, and most of the faculty were living with type 1 diabetes themselves. Diagnosed at the age of 13, Abby was the lead charge nurse at CBC and is currently a registered nurse in an endocrinologist's office, working toward her goal of becoming a certified diabetes educator (CDE). *"Having diabetes shaped my life goals in a huge way. After working at a camp specifically for kids with type 1 diabetes, I realized that I wanted to teach children about diabetes, forever, as my job. It was my passion. I went to nursing school with the intention of becoming a CDE and am currently working toward that goal. Being around kids who are growing up with diabetes presents a great opportunity for adults who have gone through that experience to help them with the hurdles they will encounter. That's what I love to do."*

Despite being driven, career-wise, by her personal experiences with diabetes, diabetes does not stand to define Abby. *"I tell everyone that, whether they have diabetes or a family member does, or even just a friend, we are people, first and foremost. I am Abby. I'm a nurse, I love yoga, and I have diabetes. It's the last detail about me, as a person, but among the most important. Diabetes is just part of my life."*

Similarly, fellow diabetes blogger Kim Vlasnik finds diabetes as a common outlet for her passions and wants to connect and give back. Like me, her vehicle became the Internet. *"Going online to find other adults living with type 1 ended up being one of the best things I've ever done for my health. The connections and camaraderie I've found in the diabetes online community help me feel less alone and isolated, and more like I'm actually a member of a really exclusive club that no one ever wants to join. Before that, diabetes was this thing, this burden I just kept to myself. Aside from a couple years of diabetes summer camp as a kid, I didn't really have a lot of contact with other kids with type 1."*

And that's it—that's totally it for me. Connecting with other people who understand this disease makes it less of a burden and less chaotic. The swirl of type 1 diabetes can go from manageable to maelstrom in a matter of minutes, and keeping things predictable in efforts to be proactive can be challenging. Finding kindred spirits and embracing the "me, too!" aspect of interacting with other people with diabetes are what keep my psychosocial health from spinning out of control, helping me accept the reality of life with diabetes, whatever it may be that day. And, keeping tabs on my emotional health helps me keep a tighter, more active rein on my physical health. For me, that is where my sense of balance exists. It's the sweet spot. (Stop groaning—I'm just getting started with these horrible diabetes puns. You just wait until we get to the chapter on making excessively sweet love.)

Briley Boisvert, diagnosed at the age of two, finds that sense of acceptance to be the root of what keeps her balanced. *"Diabetes can never be the sole focus in a person's life, whether you are the person with diabetes or the spouse, parent, or child of someone with diabetes. Life is about living, and living it to the fullest. Fill your time with a variety of things! For me, I choose family, friends, skiing, running, tennis, reading, laughing with kids, and more. Every person is different and every person needs more than one focus. The biggest thing to understand is that all of those other things can be done, but diabetes will be there also. Once you accept that, it's much easier to live."*

In my life, the balance I sought as a child is different from what I seek as an adult. When I was diagnosed with type 1 diabetes, the person in charge of my health wasn't me. It was the job of my parents. Now, for better or for worse, I am the one in charge, and I need to own all aspects of diabetes.

I'm proud and feel accomplished when I take a step forward, and equally embarrassed and critical of myself when I take a step backward. I think my biggest step forward has been sharing my story with the world through the Internet, chronicling both the forward *and* backward steps. Being able to share in a medium that allows people who understand and live with this condition in some capacity or another to comment and create a conversation has helped me to see that I'm not alone. This new, but no longer lonely, normal is something I share with so many others who survive, and inspire me to thrive, with diabetes. And in this, my first book, I want to share my personal experiences and the experiences of so many others who balance life and diabetes every day.

Chapter Two

Before and After

"At the time when I became sure that something was wrong, I was in Wyoming skiing. I had been losing weight and getting progressively weaker. My vision was often blurry, and I had an insatiable thirst, with a commensurate need to urinate. I remember a particular day when I was lapping a run that had a bathroom and a small snack shack near the bottom of the chair lift. I would use the bathroom, guzzle a Gatorade®, then ride the lift back up. By the time I reached the top of the lift, my mouth would be so dry that it would be sticking together and I would have to pee again. I would race down the hill and repeat the process," said Christopher Angell, diagnosed with type 1 diabetes at the age of 30. He is describing some of the classic symptoms of diabetes—excessive thirst and excessive urination.

"My appetite was also getting progressively more

heroic/disturbing. I would frequently eat five or six full meals per day, but never feel satisfied for long," he explained. *"One of the final straws came when I ate an entire package of hotdogs."* Pause. *"For breakfast."*

(For the record, mass hotdog consumption has yet to be added to the list of classic symptoms of diabetes.)

Type 1 diabetes isn't diagnosed only in small children. Although I was diagnosed as a child, with very little recollection of life before diabetes, many others are diagnosed later in life, well into their established adulthood. Insulin vials in the fridge? Daily injections? Blood sugar fluctuations? These have *always* been a part of my life. All of my memories, save for a precious few, are rooted in the "after." But I've often thought about what it must be like to be handed such a huge diagnosis at a time when you're already an established adult, with a crafted sense of self. What's it like to see the line in the sand, marking life before diabetes and then this new life after diagnosis? What's it like to remember and to have to move forward as a person with diabetes?

Christopher and I spoke about the definitive "before" and "after" of diabetes, as integrating diabetes into his adult life was a new and prickly beast. Literally. He described to me the very first time he gave himself an insulin injection.

"I thought that having to give myself a shot was major. I couldn't even really conceive of it. As a perfect illustration of just how poorly I understood what kind of life lay ahead of me, the first night I gave myself my Lantus® injection,

I actually set up a camera to film it. I very methodically took out the pen, opened a fresh needle, and screwed it on. I dialed up two units and pushed them out to make sure the pen was primed. Then I lifted my shirt, chose just the right spot, and wiped it thoroughly with an alcohol swab. I dialed up 15 units, and, trying to be brave but also make it clear to the camera just HOW BIG A DEAL this was, pushed the needle through my skin. I pressed the button all the way in, leaving it there for 15 seconds to get every precious drop.

I don't have the video. I had actually paused it when I thought I was pressing record, so I had videos of before and after the shot. But it didn't matter. Soon I had given myself dozens and then hundreds and then thousands of shots, and the idea of recording them quickly became ludicrous."

Manny Hernandez remembers his first low blood sugar, which happened one night while he was reading a book about diabetes and his wife was reading a book about pregnancy. *"I had been recently diagnosed. At the time, I was operating under the assumption that I had type 2 diabetes so I was reading Gretchen Becker's book about the first year with diabetes. My wife and I had also recently found out we were pregnant, so we were reading* What To Expect When You're Expecting. *We were reading the baby book in bed and had just finished a section about how husbands sometimes experience pregnancy-like symptoms. Shortly after, I felt strange. I couldn't quite put my finger on it, but it wasn't 'normal.' I told my wife and her first reaction was, 'I am sure you are just saying that because of what we just read in the pregnancy book ...' and then it dawned on her what we had read in the diabetes book about low blood sugars. She ran for the meter, and sure enough I was low—42 mg/dL."*

Sometimes the challenge for an adult diagnosed with type 1 diabetes is to make sure they get the correct diagnosis in the first place. Christopher talked about his initial diagnosis, which included the false assumption that, because of his age (30) and the fact that an in-office finger stick showed a result in the mid-300s, he had type 2 diabetes. *"They sent me home with a prescription for metformin and an Accu-Chek Aviva® meter. I was told to avoid candy or sugar, but not told anything about carbohydrates."* However, weeks later, his symptoms persisted, and he continued to lose weight.

"About two weeks after my initial diagnosis, I returned to my doctor to try something else—insulin." It wasn't until about six to eight months later that Christopher had proper blood work done, confirming a diagnosis of type 1 diabetes.

Like Christopher, many adults who have type 1 are misdiagnosed with type 2, based on assumptions that age or weight dictates the type of diabetes. But a type 1 diabetes diagnosis in adulthood is a growing concern. Many people in their 20s, 30s, and even 40s and 50s are being diagnosed with type 1, making their adjustment to diabetes even more difficult.

"I was diagnosed at age 30, as part of my regular yearly checkup," said Manny Hernandez, cofounder of the Diabetes

Hands Foundation, a nonprofit diabetes organization. He has been living with latent autoimmune diabetes in adults (LADA) since 2002. After several months of trying different treatments for type 2 diabetes without seeing significant results, Manny revisited his doctor. "*I was overweight so, when he saw an elevated fasting blood sugar, my primary care physician assumed I had type 2 diabetes. After months of trying a number of metformin-based treatments with minimal results, my doctor referred me to an endocrinologist. This time I tested positive for GAD antibodies and my c-peptide levels were low enough to make my endo conclude that I didn't have type 2 diabetes, but instead LADA. It wasn't until I started on insulin that it sank in that I actually had a chronic condition.*"

However, it's not just the methods of treatment that need to be integrated into a life with diabetes. Going from an injection-free lifestyle to needing several shots a day is a huge change, but often the physical demands of diabetes pale in comparison to the daily psychosocial change that people with diabetes face.

"*Before diabetes, I took so much for granted,*" said Manny. "*I knew life without diabetes for 30 years. I didn't really pay attention to my lifestyle and I certainly wasn't too mindful about all the things my body does on its own. It's such a humbling experience when you realize that, even with all the technology in the world, you still can't get it right every time. It reminds me of when I used to scuba dive. I re-*

member thinking about how much gear you have to wear to dive even a few feet deep, whereas a tiny fish just swims past you with nothing but his God-given body parts.

"And the change has been difficult to accept, at times. I haven't always been a person with diabetes, but I have always been a perfectionist, and with diabetes it is very hard to remain a perfectionist without becoming frustrated," said Manny, acknowledging the work that goes into having to think like a pancreas. *"It's hard to not feel frustrated even if you aren't a perfectionist. One of the biggest challenges I have had to overcome in my mind is to accept that some-times, in spite of my best efforts, I will not achieve perfection with diabetes. I try to do the best I can, every day. But the truth is, some days I do well, and some days I don't. This dis-ease is a one-day-at-a-time condition."*

Lindsay Swanson was 25 and living in Puerto Rico with her husband when she was diagnosed. *"I received a phone call a couple weeks after a routine gynecological appointment saying that my labs were abnormal, to come and pick them up, and hand deliver them to my doctor. I had a fasting blood glucose of 399 mg/dL. I didn't make it a rush, as nobody else seemed to make a big deal of it. I called my best friend, a nurse, and told her, as she was the only medical resource I had. She said, 'I think you might have diabetes, you have to go to the doctor right away.'"*

A diagnosis of diabetes rocks your world off its foundation and the learning curve is steep, but regardless of when you're diagnosed, your world does right itself. It's just different and creates an awareness of your body's mechanics and responses that were previously unacknowledged.

Lindsay agrees. *"The late-in-life diagnosis has spawned an increasing interest in total overall health and wellness, and an understanding of my body and how it works."*

People with diabetes are the original "quantified self-ers," always tracking and dealing with a demanding disease. A plate of food is never simply food, but also morphs into this complicated math problem, taking carbohydrate content and insulin:carb ratios into account. You can't just take a bite— you have to solve for X first. The urge to pee can't be just that—you also need to rule out hyperglycemia, right? The goal is for people with diabetes to do this dance while remaining true to the people we were and the people we are. But what changes when the diagnosis comes later in life? Are you still the same?

"All throughout my childhood and growing up, I always wanted to be the different one. If someone said to do something, I did the opposite. If someone stated something, I'd argue, and if someone said it couldn't be done, I'd find a way," admitted Lindsay. *"However, when I was diagnosed, it was the first time in my life when I longed to be 'normal' again and not be 'different,' which was a new and very uncomfortable position for me to be in for the first time in my life. I would say this led to initial psychosocial dysfunction, in that I was embarrassed by my type 1 diabetes and letting*

others know that I was different. I didn't want to take insulin in front of anyone, I didn't want to check my blood sugar, and I certainly didn't want to talk about it. I entered a deep depression for about a year and a half, when I truly thought my life as I knew it had come to an end.

"The most significant social impact that diabetes has on my life is that I am no longer afraid to be the new person I've become in front of others. I wasn't quite as extroverted and social before as I am now, but with type 1 diabetes being such a lonely desolate disease, the connections are lifesaving, and the only way to connect is to put yourself out there. Through these connections, I quickly learned that helping others is what empowers me most, and helps me in my own management."

"Having diabetes and immersing myself in the diabetes community have made me a more sensitive person and forced me to confront judgments that I've made in the past about other people and their health," Christopher shared, noting this as the most significant emotional change. *"I know very well that I, someone who has always been naturally skinny without doing a damn thing to get that way, would certainly judge people with type 2 differently were it not something that I learned a great deal about by virtue of living in the world of diabetes. I'm much more aware of the struggles so many people go through with their health."*

Christopher had a difficult time pinpointing where diabetes changed his life the most, as it seemed to affect a broad spectrum of experiences for him. *"It's really hard to separate diabetes into different components in terms of its impact on my life. It's such a package deal. Without meaning to sound glib, the main difference is that before diagnosis I didn't concern myself with diabetes, and now there's nothing that concerns me more. There is, with terribly few exceptions—exceptions I generally consider to be lapses on my part—no decision I make where diabetes is not considered, and many decisions that only concern diabetes. There has never been anything else in my life given that kind of primacy."*

But is balance sought? Achievable? Or just a strategy for schoolyard seesaws?

Lindsay has found some sense of balance, born from becoming part of her new tribe of people with diabetes. *"Becoming actively involved in the diabetes community in varying roles has helped me maintain balance with diabetes. It's a unique perspective when you're diagnosed with type 1 as an adult, and that created an instant passion for me to connect with others who understand. Therefore, I donate my time, money, friendship, and insight, blog, fundraise, etc. This, in turn, has provided a family of the most amazing people I've had the pleasure of meeting and getting to know. We are connected and we should be working together to support one another.*

"The life I have now is completely different than the life I had pre-diagnosis. It sounds cliché, but a good way for me

to capture this is by saying that my acceptance of the hurdles we encounter in life has been the most changed," offered Lindsay. *"I began accepting these changes as our new life. I realized they are permanent, and although I can do my best to manage my disease, I can't control it. Therefore, accepting that gave me a little bit of a release, which enabled me to be more accepting of the things that I can control, like my attitude, reactions, and the constant change that comes from living with type 1 diabetes."*

Manny admits to missing the carefree nature of life before his diabetes diagnosis, but he's found a new mission in his life, turning disease into purpose. *"I feel like I am a better and more mindful person since I became diagnosed, and I feel even more like I have a purpose in life since we started the Diabetes Hands Foundation in 2008—to bring together people touched by diabetes for positive change to make sure that nobody living with this condition ever feels alone."*

And Christopher isn't sold on the concept of balance, but instead works in pursuit of a life worth living. He said, *"I don't know that I actually seek balance. I seek health, and I want to live a long and wonderful life, but if forced to choose between the two, I'll take wonderful. I know that in order to do that, I need to work hard and make sacrifices that other people don't have to make in order to have a chance at avoiding the complications that come along with diabetes, as well as minimize the daily drags and dangers of highs and lows. And I know that even if I do an amazing job* of 'managing' my diabetes, there are no guarantees. Still, my goal is to make a life for myself that I want to live, to give myself a reason to endure everything that living with diabetes demands I endure, and then live that life. For me, that doesn't really leave room for balance. I have only one life and my life includes diabetes, so I'm going all-in with it. I sacrifice, I live, and I celebrate the life I have as best I can, and I keep trying to find new things for which I want to live. As long as I'm able to do that, I don't worry too much about balance."

Chapter Three

Transitioning from a Parent's Care to Caring for Yourself

My mom, Debbe, recalls the virus I had prior to my diabetes diagnosis, the one my endocrinologists have historically pointed to as the "trigger" that set tumbling the dominos of my diagnosis. My pediatric endocrinologist told me that my beta cells were in a ready state for type 1 diabetes, and he believed that virus is what set the wheel into motion. But the actual diagnosis? I don't really remember it much. Diabetes has always just been there.

At the hospital, the doctors and nurses spoke mostly to my parents. My dad paced the room and looked out the window. My mom sat at the table with the endocrinologist, listening and taking notes. Books on long- and short-acting insulin, a proposed diet, and a chart to log my blood sugars slid across the table. I wasn't paying too much attention to these attempts at education.

Pieces of fruit were offered to us as injection practice targets. "The skin of an orange is almost identical in strength and texture to that of human skin," the nurse said, handing a syringe to my mom along with a vial of clear solution. The tip of the syringe was thrust into the bottle to draw back a few units of saline, pretending it was insulin. The needle tip was placed easily against the side of the ripened orange and then pushed inside with little hesitation.

However, when my mother placed the tip of the needle, filled with insulin, against the fleshy part of my arm, it was not so simple. This was an intrusive change, all of these now-necessary needles, but we did what we needed to do to move forward. My mom always felt that it was important for me to learn the mechanics of this process. "*I felt that if you were more independent, you'd hopefully be less resentful of diabetes. Because it wouldn't hold you back. Independence was key,*" she explained.

This is probably why, when my childhood friend Jill had her sleepover birthday party in December, my mom made certain that I was able to attend ... even though it was only three months after my diagnosis. I packed my pajamas, my sleeping bag, my glucose meter, and my stuffed animal Kitty. I was beyond excited for my first sleepover. My mom was slightly less excited and more nervous.

Mom stayed and administered my last shot of the day, then went home, whispering that she'd be back around 6:30 the next morning to check me and give me my morning insulin. I have a clear memory of my mother and Jill's mother in the kitchen drinking tea that morning as we all wandered downstairs after our sleepover. It didn't dawn on me until later that my mother probably didn't sleep much that night, running back and forth between our house and Jill's house to monitor my newly diagnosed diabetes.

"*You did your shots pretty young, by the time you were about eight,*" my mother, Debbe, recalls. "*I would draw the insulin up and you would inject yourself. But then all of a sudden, you developed a fear of giving yourself a shot. We have no idea what caused it—no one's in your head, and you weren't telling us what your hang-up was. You just decided it was scary to pinch your skin up and put the needle in.*"

I remember these moments clearly, hiding underneath the dining room table or behind the floor-length curtains to avoid being told to take my shot. Mom was surprised at my sudden recoil.

"*I couldn't understand why you didn't want to do them, after you had already been doing them for a while,*" she shrugged as she remembered those days. "*I resumed the job of injecting but I hoped diabetes camp would reignite your interest.*"

"Clara Barton Camp for Diabetic Girls." The picture on the front of the brochure was of a smiling camp counselor and three little girls grinning and hugging each other. The background was a gorgeous lake and some cabins tucked between trees. My mom and I discussed this camp the year after I was diagnosed.

"Kerri, this camp is special. Every single camper has diabetes, like you. Every counselor has diabetes, too. I think even most of the other staff are diabetic. Everyone has it. So it's easy to go and do your tests and shots and all that stuff without worrying. Right?" She avoided making eye contact, hoping she had adequately sold me on the idea.

There were other kids with diabetes? Where the hell had they been hiding? I thought about this. A bunch of diabetic kids. I'm one of them. I'd like to meet other diabetics, so I didn't feel like I was alone. For several weeks, I was excited.

Then excitement gave way to panic as I thought about all these people I didn't know and how I was going to be living alongside them for the next two weeks. Mom and Dad drove me to camp, met my counselor and my fellow campers, chatted with a few parents, and then prepared to leave.

"Mom, I don't want to stay here." My chin trembled.

"Honey, listen. This is going to be so fun. I don't know any other kid who gets to spend part of her summer with other diabetics and having a ton of fun. Did you see the archery field? And the lake? It looked like they had a very cool arts and crafts building, too. And the dining hall is huge! I bet there will be food fights!"

I smiled a little bit, still nervous. I had no idea, though, just how nervous my parents were, giving me and responsibility for my diabetes over to this camp for almost two full weeks.

Clara Barton Camp turned out to be the most incredible experience of my young diabetic life. The campers were all diabetic, as advertised. There wasn't a person there with whom I interacted every day who wasn't also checking their blood sugar and taking their insulin shots. It had such an intense sense of community—of family—that the memories of camp still bring a smile to my face, even 20 years later.

That feeling of "normal" was a huge part of growing up with diabetes, because it kept my disease in the background instead of giving it center stage. My parents, my mother in particular, were always careful to make sure that diabetes wasn't something for which I was singled out, even though it was still on their minds.

"The fact that you went to Clara Barton Camp from the time you were diagnosed until you were too old was a blessing in that I was able to hand over the responsibility of your medical care to a very capable and trusted staff. I looked at sending you to camp as a benefit to everyone in our family. You could bond with children who dealt with the same issues you did on a daily basis. You guys could complain about how over-protective your parents were and that we don't understand what it's like.

"Because it's true—we don't understand what it's like for you. But as a parent, my children don't understand the fear that is ever-present in our minds. Will we handle their

diabetes care well enough to ensure that they don't have serious lows or highs? Have we done enough to protect their future health from diabetes complications? Have we given them the confidence to deal with complications, should they arise? It's a scary ride that we parents are on."

Learning to think and act like a pancreas was a learning curve for my parents, but passing along the torch of care to me was another journey entirely. Growing up as a kid with diabetes, my need and instinctual inclination toward independence served me well, but taking full responsibility for my diabetes management was a long and piecemeal process. Drawing up and administering my own injections was a huge step forward, as was checking my blood sugar and making decisions on how to act on the number on the meter. Driving was also a big step toward independence and diabetes self-management for me and for my parents.

My mother concurred. *"Driving was a huge turning point. It was a reward for being conscientious about diabetes. It wasn't just for your sake, but for the sake of everyone else on the road. The point was, you had this disease and you had to own it. If you didn't check before driving, then we weren't going to let you drive. You don't punish for diabetes, you punish for irresponsibility. Diabetes just happens to be an example of something to be irresponsible with."*

My mother always protected me. She and my father tried so hard and, in retrospect, I can't imagine what it was like for them to raise a child with diabetes. If tight control is a guilt-inducing component for the person with diabetes, the guilt of the parent must have the potential to be suffocating. I love my parents and believe that the reason I am secure in myself is because they instilled me with the confidence that, no matter what, my life would be good. I would come to the very end and feel like I hadn't missed a damn thing.

We didn't fight about the things my friends fought their parents over, but so many arguments were had around diabetes. My friends fought with their parents and compared battle stories over sandwiches their mothers had made them for lunch, but I never shared my tales. How was I supposed to explain to my classmates that my mother and I had a huge screaming match over my blood sugar of 385 mg/dL? How to describe the guilt I felt for eating those cupcakes and how she found the wrapper, but I refused to fess up?

"Just admit that you ate it! Just admit it!"

Defiant, I crossed my arms over my chest and stared back at her. "No! I didn't eat it!" The last bitter tastes of chocolate in my mouth stung like bees.

"Kerri, I know you did! You did! I found the wrapper!" She held it over her head triumphantly. *"I found it and you're lying! We work so hard at this—you need to be more careful."*

"*We*? We work so hard?" I started to cry but held it in as best I could and shot her a steely glance. "You don't do anything. Diabetes is *my* disease."

Frustrated, under-appreciated, and heartbroken, my mother

reeled back her foot and kicked the thing closest to her—a blue plastic bin that held my shoes underneath the bed. Her foot went through the side and left a gaping hole.

I gasped. Mom wasn't one for violence. She never spanked us. Maybe she should have, but she didn't. She gasped, too. Her foot was stuck in the wall of the blue bin and she had to lean over to wrestle it free.

"*I don't do this to hurt you,*" she said quietly, still working to free her ankle. "*I know it's not my disease. I just wish it wasn't yours.*"

We stared at each other for a minute.

"I ate the cupcakes."

"*I know you did.*"

"And I don't care that I'm high."

Sigh. "*I wish you did.*"

She stood thoughtfully for a minute, and then tossed the cupcake wrapper into my trash can. The crinkle of cellophane was the soundtrack of my guilt.

"*For now, I'll care enough for us both.*"

Another battle ended. Too hard to explain to my friends. So while they complained about breaking curfew and arguing about which boys they were allowed to date, I kept the confrontations between my mother and me private. We were fighting about what foods I was allowed to eat. But at the same time, we were fighting for my life. Passing that torch of care from her to me was one of the toughest transitions in my life with diabetes.

But, it made us close. Close in ways that mothers and daughters might not often be close. As their children, we understand on some level how hard they worked to care for us for the nine months before we came crashing into this world. But living every day watching her try to keep me safest and healthiest, it tethered me like an emotional umbilical cord. Even now, as I live states away and she's not the keeper of my diabetes management anymore, if I don't answer the phone in the morning, she worries. She always worries, some times more quietly than others and sometimes bravely out loud.

"*You have to stop being afraid of letting them* [children with diabetes] *have some control. Because you can't control it, or them, forever,*" Debbe said. "*It has to be a gradual process. It scares you, but it's their life, and eventually you have to let them decide the quality of their own life. We didn't want your life to be so safe that it was boring. You have diabetes, but you still get to live. And, as your mom, I had to trust that you could do this. I had to trust you, and trust that I did my best. So I had to let you go.*"

Chapter Four

Siblings

I don't have a clear recollection of life immediately after diagnosis, but I know back in 1986, food choices ruled the roosts of diabetes households. Once the vials of insulin moved into our refrigerator's butter compartment, gone were the Twinkies and Ring Dings and Yodels (and other snack foods comprised of a half gram of actual nutrients and then a whole pile of rubbish). Our eating patterns changed as a family, and Diet Pepsi and food scales replaced the snack cupboard of days gone by. My mother hid the ice cream sandwiches in the hollowed-out box of broccoli in the freezer. She had packages of E.L. Fudge cookies hidden between the sweaters stacked in her closet. She was a food-hoarding squirrel, with delicious treats in every obscure corner.

I viewed this as a clever approach that removed a lot of temptation (and also presented some very furtive treasure hunts with tasty rewards), and one that helped to keep me safe and healthy. But for my brother and sister, both with perfectly capable pancreases, the lifestyle change wasn't necessary. Didn't they get to have snacks, still? (My brother confirmed that he, too, was searching for the "good snacks" after my diagnosis. *"I had to look in the freezer for cookies and above the broom closet for the special sugary cereals,"* he said.)

What I failed to realize then is that my diabetes didn't have to be my siblings' diabetes. There was so much about their lives as the siblings of a child with diabetes that I couldn't even wrap my head around. I didn't know what it was like to have your sister come home from the hospital, now playing host to something no one could see, and garner so much attention (for better or for worse). I've talked to some siblings of kids with diabetes and heard about the guilt. "I felt bad for wishing I was sick, too, because I was jealous of the attention." Or the worry. "Was I going to get diabetes, too?" Or the anger. "I am sick of her diabetes being the sole focus of our family." Or, just plain fear. "Will diabetes hurt my sibling?"

My brother, Darrell, was 13 when I was diagnosed with diabetes, and old enough to remember some of the details that I can't recall. *"I remember Dr. L [our pediatrician] coming out of his office, the one with the patterned wallpaper that had giraffes and monkeys on it, and he was holding a little plastic cup with what was your urine sample. We had both gone for checkups on the same day. He told Mom that he wanted to do some additional testing for you, so Mom dropped me off at soccer practice and proceeded to take you somewhere for tests.*

"*I remember being picked up from soccer practice and leaning through the open passenger-side window. You were in the back, dressed in a little white knit pom-pom hat and looking rather dour. You looked very small to me. I believe it was there that Mom told me what the verdict was, before I even got into the car. Seeing what type of memory it has indelibly put on my mind, whether it's truly accurate or embellished by the passing of time, I knew it was something major. I knew it was a 'difficult time,' and it burned right in.*"

My little sister, Courtney, was only five when I was diagnosed, so as far as she is concerned, I've always had diabetes. "*I was so little when I found out that you were diagnosed with diabetes. All I remember is Mom and Dad telling me that you were sick. I didn't know what diabetes was until I was a little bit older, and could understand better. At that time, they told me that you had to check your blood sugar and then get a shot. I thought it was an allergy shot,*" she said, remembering her own experiences as a kid with severe allergies. "*But Mom said it different, that you were injecting a special medicine called 'insulin.'*"

Laura Watson was in fifth grade when her sister, Jacquie, was diagnosed. "*I was in the fifth grade; Jacquie was in the seventh. It was fall. My mom was encouraging Jacquie to eat as much as possible because of recent and dramatic weight loss. I remember standing in the pharmacy section of the local grocery store with my mom to pick up ketone strips. Shortly thereafter, Jacquie was just kind of gone and I got updates through my parents. A lot of what I remember about those updates involved oranges and syringes and reassurances that Jacquie was going to be okay. That year in school I had all the same teachers Jacquie had two years before. It was their reaction to the news of the diagnosis that made me realize what a big deal it was."*

My brother did realize that diabetes was something "big," but at the same time, it wasn't a topic of much discussion. *"We have only talked about things that impacted you negatively, like when there was a setback or an issue. I don't believe we've ever had a long, positive conversation, where you got a new pump or you had a good checkup."*

Like Darrell, Laura's memories of growing up alongside a sibling with diabetes weren't rooted in deep discussions and serious chats about disease management and its influence. *"I don't remember it being an intrusive force, but I don't think I filed it under 'no big deal' either. Rather, it always seemed to be something that Jacquie had under control, even if it meant a lot of work to keep it under control. I suppose I always assumed that my big sister knew what she was doing no matter what she was doing. Whether it was a decision to perm her hair, tight roll her jeans, or give herself an injection where and when, I applied the 'big sister' rule.*

"*I surely remember Jacquie having lows and highs and in some cases being exhausted the next day from a middle-of-the-night low,*" added Laura, recalling these moments. "*If there were cereal bowls and/or almost-empty Coke cans around when I got up in the morning, I could usually guess that Jacquie would be sleeping in.*"

Darrell also had memories of my hypoglycemic aftermath, with only one clear memory of watching me in the midst of a low. "*There were moments of fear, as I once was with you during a low and you told me that you saw car headlights coming out of your hands if you held them up to your face, like cars racing toward you on a dark highway. I had nothing to compare it to, so that was frightening.*"

Funny thing is, I remember that symptom. When I was a little kid, my hypoglycemic experiences were very heady and confusing. I distinctly remember many lows where I'd see things, borderline hallucinations, and my fear of them was all-consuming. One time, while our babysitter Kim was watching my brother, sister, and me, I remember sitting in the hallway with my back against the wall, screaming about those cars coming out of my hands. I remember the headlights zooming toward me, and a panicky feeling that I would be hit by these cars. It was irrational, but my brain was shifting the glucose reserves around, preserving the parts of my brain that were necessary for autonomic processes, such as breathing and the beating of my heart. Rationale fell by the wayside as my body tried to make sense without enough glucose in my cells.

As bizarre as this feeling was to experience, I at least had an idea of when it was starting, and felt the relief when it began to end. My brother and sister were left just to watch and wonder what the hell was happening.

"*I think the strongest impact that diabetes has had on you is that you became very aware of your own mortality at a very, very early age. Here was something that had, and always will have, the potential of taking years from you, or your life itself if it's not managed properly. It's an everyday cumulative tightrope,*" said Darrell, when asked about how diabetes has affected our relationship. "*Some people would take that and internalize it, where you took it and swung the momentum into a force of motivation. Your siblings know how you think, being the closest thing to a 'twin,' and even though I know you are absolutely terrified at times, you'll still face it head on.*"

I also spoke with Jackie Singer, the twin sister of Mollie Singer, who lives with type 1 diabetes. "*When Mollie was diagnosed, it was as if I was diagnosed, and our whole family was diagnosed,*" she said. "*We really did live, breathe, and eat as a family and that meant doing what Mollie could do when Mollie could do it. I never really worried about becoming diabetic, but there were many times when I wish I was, because then she wouldn't have to go through what she had to go through by herself.*

"*Mollie and I were inseparable before she was diagnosed and we are the same way now, if not closer. When we were in school, we had all the same classes from kindergarten through college. I was as knowledgeable as her about diabetes, so I was always by her side in case of an emergency. When we were little, we always shared a bedroom and there were so many nights I would stay awake to make sure she was okay. It was terrifying to think that one morning I would wake up and she wouldn't. I became her protector, always aware of changes in her breathing or sleeping, setting alarms to remind her to check her blood sugar at the appropriate time, grabbing juice and a snack for her when she couldn't, and on two occasions before we were ten years old, setting up the glucagon kit and calling 911 while our mom held Mollie in her arms after she experienced an episode with dangerously low blood sugar levels."*

Diabetes is a disease that affects the whole family. It's not just the person who is receiving the injections or pump infusion sets or finger pricks who's carrying the full weight of diabetes. I don't know if my brother and sister understood what diabetes meant when I was first diagnosed and if any of us understood just how big the words *without a cure* really were. But I know that we learned about diabetes as a family, and dealt with it the same way.

There is that dance that occurs between my brother and sister and me, that weird discussion that never really takes place, where siblings acknowledge that there is something serious in play, but no one wants to talk about it so plainly. We didn't sit around the breakfast table and run commentary on the state of my fasting blood sugars, but diabetes was always present and always somewhere on the table, literally and figuratively. If it wasn't my mother telling me to eat all of my breakfast because I already took insulin for it, it was her reminding me to grab my lunch bag.

There was a time—only once—when I felt angry. Jealous of my healthy brother and sister and the fact that their days didn't start and end with needles. I was about 14 years old and pouring out my angst into a fabric-bound journal, scribbling in it madly with a ball point pen.

"*They* don't have to worry. I'm jealous of that. But I'm worried. I'm worried about what my body will be like in like two decades, after all that time with diabetes."

I thought I was alone in that worry. It wasn't until I was deeply immersed in sharing my diabetes life with the Internet that I truly grasped how much my older brother watched and understood.

In May 2005, my first evidence of diabetic eye disease started to show in the form of cotton wool spots. Noticed during my yearly dilated eye exam, the doctor saw a few spots of swelling of the surface layer of the retina, when a part of the eye isn't provided with enough oxygen due to a damaged blood vessel. On the photos of my retina, it looked like puffy spider webs had taken up residence in my eyes.

Trying to acknowledge and understand this first diabetes-related complication, I wrote a blog post about the experience of "finding out," and explained this new situation as best I could, while trying to remain positive. Folks who were reading my blog at the time left very kind, supportive comments and their words soothed me, reminding me that this wasn't "the beginning." But it was the comment my brother left that cracked the concept of complications wide open for me, assuring me that there was life to be found after this diagnosis, too. And I'd better damn well seize it.

He wrote: "*When we were little in stature, the snow would cover our backyard like a puffy comforter. We would go out into the backyard to build snow forts, to go sledding, and to eat a majority of it. We also had this thing where we would try to go as long as possible without damaging the 'virgin' snow, keeping to our trails and cordoned off zones, in an attempt to stave off ruin. We were a prepubescent Snow-Peace, minus the trademark galleon. It would only last for so long, before the snow would melt, no matter how hard we tried to preserve it with the no-walk, no-eat zones, but we knew there'd be more snow to cover up the previous damage we had done. You've done so well, for so very long. The way you think and operate, I see a snowscape for you for a very long time ... just don't forget to eat some snow once in a while.*"

Diabetes isn't just a balancing act for the people living with it, but the people living near it and caring for people with it. I never knew that my brother noticed what I did to take care of my diabetes, and I hadn't thought ahead to how he would be impacted by any future issues. He wasn't feeling the highs and lows, but he saw them and they left an imprint on him, too. Now that my brother has two children of his own, he's mentioned that diabetes is on his radar as a parent, not just as a sibling. "*I can't help but think that it was the simple roll of the genetic dice. I keep tabs on my children's weight and how many ounces of fluids they drink as opposed to how often they go to the bathroom,*" he admitted, when I asked him about watching my niece and nephew for possible symptoms.

My sister agreed, confirming that my diabetes was an ever-present force, but something that lived on the periphery of our lives. "*Diabetes didn't really affect my childhood. There were food changes that Darrell and I had to adapt to, with a lot of the sugary foods we used to eat being cut out. Lucky Charms cereal was replaced by Cheerios. Regular lemonade was replaced by that Crystal Light stuff. We still ran around the house, though, and got into trouble. Picked on one an-other. Diabetes didn't really change much, in that sense.*"

Laura found herself in a similar situation as a sister, focusing on the hard-to-pinpoint effect that diabetes may have had on her life. "*I don't feel it's had an effect, but maybe that's how it's had an effect. Maybe Jacquie wishes that it were more front and center for me, or that I would have been more helpful when we were younger. She was kind enough to participate in a Science Fair Project for me in the tenth grade. She was my only participant. I basically made her check her blood sugar, jump on the exercycle that was in our kitchen, and check her blood sugar again. I made it to the State Science Fair that year and was placed next to participants who were proposing cures for cancer and ways to reduce the spread of oil in the event of an oil spill. I was surprised because, to me, it seemed I was just presenting a day in the life of my sister and her blood sugar levels. It wasn't until we started to spend more time together as adults—even if just on vacation—that I feel I'm really understanding what a burden she's been carrying around."*

So what do you do, if you're the sibling of a person with diabetes? It's not your disease to manage, but it resides in a person about whom you care deeply, so it becomes yours, in a sense. Jackie found that she could make the biggest impact, and be the best supporter for her sister, simply by being there for Mollie. *"The comfort of knowing they're not alone and that there's someone who's got their back no matter what makes their struggles a little easier to bear. Sometimes that's all anyone needs to help them get through the day. For someone with diabetes, it's always one day at a time."*

Laura and my siblings agreed with Jackie, but also mentioned the need to be there for the moments of acute need, such as low blood sugars. *"I don't know if it's best to make a big deal out of it or to try to make life seem more normal by not making a big deal out of it,"* said Laura. *"All I knew to do was to be there with a juice box, if needed."*

Darrell concurred. *"Be ready to help if a low or high occurs, as I know your greatest fear is to have that happen alone, with no one to assist when your body and mind aren't cooperating. Young siblings should know how to call 911 and/or parents if there are issues. Other than that, treat them no differently. There's so much change and so many routines a person with diabetes has to do to work to be healthy, I'm sure they'd appreciate just being a brother or sister to them."*

He added, *"That and look beneath the frozen snap peas for the M&Ms."*

Chapter Five

Weaving the Threads of Friendship and Diabetes

It was fifth grade and Mrs. Latimer was my language arts teacher. It was the first year I'd ever had a locker and they were strategically located outside of the language arts classroom. Being totally honest, I felt wicked cool having a locker. It was such a rite of passage, to the point where I actually cut out pictures from a *Tiger Beat* magazine and hung them inside of the door. (Isn't that what you were supposed to do, in fifth grade? Like it was some after-school special on Nickelodeon?) Nicole, my locker partner, and I cut out pictures of tropical fish and fashioned a pretend aquarium out of the locker—we went so far as to make a fake filter out of a used water bottle and some aluminum foil.

One day as two of my friends and I walked back from the cafeteria after lunch, we stopped by our lockers to toss in our lunch bags. Christie grabbed her reading book from the top shelf of her locker. Nicole didn't need anything because she already had her book. I reached into the bottom of our locker to retrieve a reading book and saw a folded up piece of paper stuck in the locker vents.

"To Kerri Only."

A note! I got a note! Fifth-grade immaturity gave way to giggles and blushing as we crowded around the note to read.

"Dear Kerri, the Dirty Diabetic. No one likes you. We've made a whole club about how we don't like you. It's called the We Hate Diabetics Club." A picture of a needle encased in an accusatory red circle was scribbled beside my name.

Nicole and Christie stood there, not saying anything. I started to cry.

Through the miraculous methods that only fifth-grade language arts teachers possess, Mrs. Latimer found out who had left that note in the locker. The We Hate Diabetics Club consisted of one redheaded girl who sat with me at lunch, whose eyes were red rimmed as she shuffled, with the urging of Mrs. Latimer's hands, toward me to say that she was sorry.

There are enormous parts of my childhood that I remember in great detail—the wild organ music that sprang forth from the Flying Horses Carousel in Watch Hill. Fishing off the dock at the summer house, catching nothing more than trouble for standing too close to the edge of the mooring. My childhood was dribble sandcastles at the town beach during the summer and sprawling sand villages at Napatree Point in the snow of winter. I remember skinning my knee when

I fell off my bike in my own driveway, only to ride all the way to the neighbor's house to have the kiss and the Band-Aid applied.

These are the things I remember. My childhood is painted in vivid colors and is hardly touched by diabetes, for the most part. But there are moments that I remember feeling very, very diabetic. Like that moment with the redheaded girl in fifth grade who started her little club.

Kids are mean, and if it wasn't diabetes for which they were picking on me, it would have been something else. Kids have a way of preying on those who are perceived as different. But in my experiences, diabetes was a difference that helped me find my self-confidence footing and gave me a reason to have to stand up for myself. Part of that meant finding, and keeping, friends who were worth my time.

The mountain of learning that comes as part of a close friendship with a person who has type 1 diabetes isn't hard to climb, when you're dedicated. As a little kid, my friends had diabetes explained to them by way of their parents, who had diabetes explained to them by my mom. Every new friendship I made in elementary school came with my mom visiting the parents of my new friend, to fill them in on what diabetes meant and how they could help keep me safest.

As I grew older, I took that theme of disclosure and applied it liberally. My friend Julie wasn't the only friend I had who found a sudden stash of flattened granola bars in their purses, or test strips in weird places.

"*Kerri, I found a test strip in the brand new car I bought last week. Brand new,*" read a text message from her. "*You haven't even been in this car yet!*"

"*I didn't know too much about diabetes prior to us living together in college,*" said Heidi, who was one of my roommates. "*When we moved in together our junior year of college, I do remember being really interested in your diabetes devices and what you had to do every day to manage type 1 diabetes. Remember when we'd go grocery shopping, all seven of us, and spend like $500? We always bought sugar-free jam for you. I learned that salad wasn't going to have a serious effect on you, but ice cream or regular jam could cause a blood sugar problem.*"

Heidi also brought up the meeting I had with my roommates, when we all moved into a house together for the school year. "*When we first moved into our house, you had a conversation with us all about diabetes and what to do if you ever needed the glucagon.*" I remember that, too. It was a strange combination of trying to alleviate my own fears while trying not to scare my friends, but in the end, we all felt safer knowing there was a plan for a worst-case scenario. Once that plan was established, we moved on, having an incredibly fun time at college.

My best friend, Lynnae, and I met when I was midway through college. I was looking for a summer job and wanted to find a fun, active waitressing job down by the beach near where I lived. I had been working at a catering place earlier in the year, but after a slip-and-fall accident involving large catering trays and breaking my tailbone (true, and painful, story), I needed a lower-impact employment opportunity while my butt healed.

I applied at a breakfast restaurant that happened to be owned by Lynnae's parents. I walked in, intending to march confidently over to the register and ask if they were hiring, but instead, the swinging door bonked me on my injured tailbone just after I entered the room, forcing me to awkwardly yell ouch as the heavy door smacked against me. Everyone stopped to look at me and I died slowly of embarrassment.

"Hi. I'm hoping you guys are hiring? Sorry about yelling. I broke my butt recently."

I was hired immediately. And soon thereafter, I befriended the owner's daughter, who has since become my closest friend (and subsequently my maid of honor, and then the god-mother of my daughter).

Diabetes was an easy discussion with Lynnae, as both of her parents have type 2 diabetes. Disclosure came in the form of telling my boss—her mother—and sharing that, if my blood sugar became low while working, I may need to grab some orange juice or glucose tabs during my shift. "Oh, I feel you, honey," she said. "I have lows sometimes, too. I get sweaty when I'm low. Here," she said, showing me a hairdryer that she kept underneath the counter in the staff bathroom. "If you need this, feel free to use it."

Everyone on staff understood my diabetes as much as they

needed to, and I spent the summer slinging eggs, pouring coffee, and occasionally ducking into the staff bathroom to blow-dry my hypoglycemia-dampened head.

"I never thought of you as my diabetic friend. You're Kerri, who happens to have diabetes," Lynnae told me over coffee, as our daughters tore through my house dressed as Batman and a ballerina. *"But I did spy on your blood sugars. I know you don't ignore those numbers, but if you were going low, I was prepared. I needed to be prepared."*

Now, years later as a healthcare professional, Lynnae sees diabetes in all of its forms. She sees the newly diagnosed patient come through the hospital, confused about the language of diabetes and the implications of those words on their life. She sees the established patient come through showing evidence of diabetes-related complications, with a side of diabetes-induced guilt. She sees people who are struggling, and part of her role as both a healthcare professional and a personal diabetes caregiver is to help patients put their diabetes into context. *"I'm not talking with them about their numbers in a way that blames them, but I want to help them put the pieces of their lives together in a way that improves their health. If I can connect with what's going on in their life, then I can connect with the person and hopefully help.*

"But it is different when it's you. Or when it's my mom, or dad. You guys are my family, and seeing you struggle is so different from seeing patients that I barely know. Sometimes I feel less like a healthcare professional and more like a nag,"

she admitted. "*I want to go into my parents' house and just clean all of the cookies and candy out of it. I want to protect them, you know? But when I see what I see at work, I feel like the girl who knows too much when it comes to type 2 diabetes. I don't see a lot of type 1 diabetes at work, though. With you, it's sometimes like I don't know enough.*"

I thought about the times when Lynnae would visit me at college, coming out with my roommates and me for a night out. "*I remember one time, in particular, when you were drinking and you also had a low blood sugar. It wasn't an emergency, but juice was a faster option than the snacks you had in your bag,*" she said.

"Is that when you jumped behind the bar to grab an orange juice from the bartender?" I asked.

"*Yes. I was afraid if I asked him for juice, it would come with vodka in it or something, or a ton of ice. I needed orange juice, straight up!*"

That's the crux of the diabetes that Lynnae sees, the needing juice, or maybe the going-to-the-doctor part of it. She sees my pump when we're at the beach, and she hears my continuous glucose monitor (CGM) wail when my numbers are out of target range. She sees me trying, and failing, and succeeding, sometimes all in the same moment.

One winter afternoon, just after I had moved into a new place and had spent the afternoon unpacking boxes and putting up shelves, I had a severe hypoglycemic reaction. One of the worst I've ever had. It came sneaking up on me and scooped me up like a trap set in the woods for wild game. While the memory of the moment itself is heavy with fog (as most low memories are), I remember sitting on the floor in front of my refrigerator, a carton of orange juice next to me and phone in hand. Lynnae remembers more details, though.

"*You called me when you were low, remember? You weren't making much sense, but you kept saying, 'I'm really low and I just want you to know I'm low, just in case. Just in case. Because I'm really low, but I had juice.' I wanted to get into my car immediately and drive over there, but you kept insisting you were okay. And I realized you would be, but it was the longest few minutes ever, waiting for you to return to your voice, you know?*"

This is what most of my friends see, these parts of diabetes that make themselves known so briefly and then go back into hiding. But my closest friends are the ones who see past the brevity of a frustrating hypoglycemic moment. They're the ones who understand how this disease makes my brain a tangled mess at times, and they help pick the knots.

I was exactly two and a half weeks pregnant when I called Lynnae to share my news, the news I could barely keep from her even another minute. You see, she was four and a half months pregnant with her own child.

The scream she let out when I told her the news almost shattered my eardrum, and I'm fairly certain it damaged the speaker on my phone. And months later, when she came to the hospital to meet my daughter—her goddaughter—for the first time, it was a moment happily burned into my memory forever.

Diabetes wasn't ever a driving force behind our friendship, but as my best friend, she has taken responsibility for my health and wellness even in moments where I wouldn't have thought, or dared, to ask.

"I was prepared to carry a baby for you, you know," she told me the other night. *"I know diabetes and pregnancy and all the stuff that comes with it was something you were scared of. I even talked with [her husband] about it. I knew becoming a mom was what you wanted most, and my family was ready to help you have your family."*

She's played an instrumental part in my health and well-being up to this point. She thinks about my diabetes in a way that only my parents and husband can truly understand. Never once did she question whether our friendship was worth investing in, due to diabetes, because she knew that my health would be best if my network had her in it. Her support and friendship have brought me to this point in my life where I can live well with diabetes and enjoy the chaos of parenthood. And now she's the godmother of my most favorite person in the world—my daughter.

If that's not coming full circle, I don't know what is.

Chapter Six

Diabetes and Pregnancy

Growing up, I didn't have fantasies about the wedding with the white dress and the table seating charts and the guest list. I hoped I would end up with a partner who loved me and treated me well, and thankfully, I did find that person.

While I didn't dream about my wedding, I've always dreamt about being a mom. It was different than the dreams I had of being a writer and a race car driver (tasks never performed simultaneously, though). My dreams of motherhood were always a little cloudy, veiled in the insecurity of what a pregnancy with diabetes would be like. Doctors told my mother for years—immediately upon diagnosis, actually—that women with diabetes, particularly those diagnosed when they were really young, would have a tougher time getting pregnant and seeing the pregnancy through. I pretended not to hear them, but their words settled in my head and I was always hopeful, but never sure, that a baby would become part of my life.

I was raised to view diabetes as the most important factor in planning my pregnancy, which is why my husband and I started thinking about our future children at the same time we were planning our wedding. Historically, my A1C test results (a measure of average blood sugar levels over a span of time rather than at a specific point in time) always struggled to stay at the 7% range, and I knew it was going to take some dedication to bring my control to a point where a "healthy baby range" A1C wasn't the product of too many low blood sugars. So while we picked out wedding cake and decided on a honeymoon destination, I was already planning for our future baby.

Melissa Baland Lee, diagnosed with type 1 at the age of ten, spoke about her struggle for that target A1C. "*My husband and I were married in late 2007 and we wanted children immediately, but my A1C had never been below 7%. I wanted to be pregnant and I wanted it right away. My endocrinologist and my CDE were onboard with aggressively bringing my diabetes management into baby-making range, but they were adamant that my A1C come down to near 6%. My CDE said we should treat my management as though I were 'already pregnant, and then all we add is the baby.'*"

"*Diabetes was the main factor in the pregnancy planning process,*" asserts Lindsay Rhoades, diagnosed with type 1 diabetes just before she turned 27. *"I've always been a yo-yo'er with my management, and my endo wanted me to have three consistently improving A1C results, all with a 7% or under goal before giving me the 'green light' to try for a baby."*

Karen Hoffman was diagnosed with type 1 diabetes at the age of 15 and was raised with the same view of pregnancy as me. *"I honestly never thought I'd be able to have biological children. I was diagnosed shortly after the Diabetes Control and Complications Trial (DCCT) ended in 1993—not exactly the diabetes dark ages, but nothing like where we are today. And back then, I was essentially told that kids weren't in the cards for me—as an impressionable teenager, that notion stuck. But the years passed, tech got better, research got better, and my husband and I realized we were using outdated information. I was terrified, but I decided it could be done with hard work and a good medical team. So diabetes was a huge factor in the planning process. I got a recommendation for a high-risk obstetrician (OB) from my endo—I wanted to be sure she'd worked with type 1s before—and saw the OB for a preconception consultation. I had my eyes and heart checked to make sure I'd be safe; I started wearing a pump for the first time in my life; I logged and e-mailed my doctors and worked and worked and worked to get my A1C down below 6.0 for the first time since I was in high school. Diabetes was probably the biggest factor in the planning process. We both felt a little shocked once we got the green light to actually think about the getting pregnant part of the process.*"

After talking with several other women with diabetes who have experienced a pregnancy, I saw this theme of needing to be "green lit" or "approved" for pregnancy. I remember being petrified, during the course of bringing my A1C into baby range, of becoming pregnant without being in that range yet. The pressure for any mother-to-be to do everything "right" for their child is intense, and adding diabetes to the list of things to take into account is a loaded deck, for sure. It becomes the thing you can blame for everything. ("She burped during the ultrasound? Surely that's because I have diabetes, right?") Being able to think ahead about pregnancy does help, but it doesn't remove all the variables.

And not all pregnancies happen on the heels of an intense planning session. "*Because of the old type 1 diabetes and other health issues, I didn't even expect to get pregnant, and when I did, I was terrified,*" said Jacquie Wojick, type 1 since the age of 12 and the mother of a healthy, almost-one-year-old. "*I knew there was a good possibility I would be okay, but I also heard a lot of scary things from my doctors concerning my health and the health of my child. There's a long list of complications that children of type 1 moms are more prone to, and then there was everything else—my age, the fact that I was taking antidepressants, and pre-pregnancy alcohol consumption.*"

Neither can every pregnancy difficulty be traced back to,

and blamed on, diabetes. *"I was cleared to try to conceive and then assumed it would happen instantly. I started using a CGM, too, which helped me stay at 6.1% over the eight maddening months it took for me to actually get pregnant,"* shared Melissa. *"After several months of trying to conceive, I made an appointment with a reproductive endocrinologist. Tests revealed nothing to be concerned about. We just were among the 10 to 20 percent of couples who weren't pregnant yet after that long, and we conceived our daughter after a cycle of Clomid and an injected ovulatory stimulant. Diabetes had taken up so much attention on my radar that infertility concerns had never crossed my mind!"*

Dads with diabetes also need to consider their health status when preparing for pregnancy, despite the fact that they are not the ones who are actually pregnant. Sean Oser, living with type 1 for 24 years and the father of twin girls, remembers being given some unsolicited advice from his doctor, after he had just proposed to his now-wife. *"Tamara [Sean's wife] had gamely come along with me for a routine appointment. After our usual chat, exam, and data review, the doctor then invited both of us back to his private office, where he suddenly explained that our children would have twice the likelihood of developing type 1 diabetes because I have it, and that the background 1 percent risk doubled would therefore be 2 percent. Neither of us was ready to even think about having kids—we had just gotten engaged."*

Before our daughter joined our family, I did a lot of

research about pregnancy with diabetes. Hard facts, statistics, and professional recommendations were available by the fistful. The problem was finding anecdotal information about managing pregnancy and diabetes at the same time. Before my husband and I started trying for a baby, I felt prepared. I was worried that it would take months for us to get pregnant, but we had the blessing of a pregnancy in our first month of trying. Actually, we found out at a routine checkup at the pregnancy clinic. Those two pink lines on the pregnancy test caused me to gasp, and the certified diabetes educator clapped excitedly and exclaimed, "We never get to tell people! They usually come in to tell us!" And suddenly, I wanted nothing more than to find a room full of other pregnant women who had diabetes, so I could immerse myself in their support and say, "I have NO CLUE what I'm doing!! HELP!!"

Thing is, most pregnancy discussions don't take that kind of personal turn. I'd attended a few pre-pregnancy support groups, and I remember leaving with panic in my stomach and a lack of eyelids because I was so bugged out about the information that was presented. Pregnancy isn't easy, even if you take diabetes out of the equation, so being pelted with gobs of information on "what to expect" can be completely overwhelming. For me, it made me scared to try and unsure if I could actually do it successfully.

(I refused to open this chapter with a reference to *Steel Magnolias*, but it must be brought up now that we're all the way in here.) When I was diagnosed with type 1 diabetes, the movie *Steel Magnolias* was the mainstream example of a pregnancy with type 1 diabetes. The main character in the movie has type 1 diabetes and—spoiler alert—she dies soon after giving birth to her son. There are some amazing performances in that film, but still, not the best imagery for a young girl with diabetes. This is precisely why women sharing their stories of pregnancy with diabetes were and are so important to me. Their stories—our stories—of real-life diabetic pregnancies are what movies should be based on. Nice, mundane, nothing-out-of-the-ordinary-happens sort of movies.

Is there a balance to be struck with pregnancy and diabetes as we work our way through the nine months? Can we, as women with diabetes, achieve the pregnancy goal of "run of the mill?"

Karen went through one pregnancy two years ago and is currently building baby No. 2. *"Balance? Oh, that was—and is now—an incredibly hard thing. Hard enough, in fact, that I think I kind of picked a priority. It sounds weird, but I just let my body do its own thing for the pregnancy. I went to the appointments, let the doctors do their thing, read all the books, but I was just incredibly focused on my diabetes— it was my number-one time spend. The logging, the food weighing, the e-mailing with my team, the testing and set changing, the emotional upheavals and stress and all those time-consuming parts of diabetes became the things that I focused on—and experienced—the most. Everything took a* backseat to diabetes. It didn't make for a joyful pregnancy, but it was the way I coped with my fears about being pregnant and diabetic.

"Things are a lot different with my current pregnancy, though, partly because I'm more relaxed about diabetes and partly because I'm not balancing time with just diabetes, pregnancy, and work—I've also got a toddler in the mix. That's actually the hardest part of this pregnancy. I feel like I don't have enough hours in the day—or, frankly, the energy—to give 100 percent to both of my kids. I think my daughter gets a less-awesome mom than she should, but I take comfort from the fact that she has a huge, loving heart and is absolutely the kind of person who would understand that sometimes mama needs to take care of herself or her brother first before she can have playtime or a dance party."

For many women with diabetes, the extra appointments and exams that come with a pregnancy that is deemed "high risk" can be a tough topic to handle at work. Jacquie was grateful that time off wasn't an issue for her. "I'm lucky to work at a place that was flexible with my schedule, so I was able to take time off of work. If I didn't have the support of my husband and my workplace, or the health insurance I did, I don't know what I would have done. I will say that I found being pregnant with diabetes to be one of the most emotionally exhausting things I have ever experienced. I hated it. In fact, I can't really say I balanced it at all; I spent a lot of time feeling sorry for myself. I also slept a lot, since it was one of *the few things I could do that wouldn't mess with my blood sugar."*

Lindsay let her employer know about her pregnancy right away, to help manage time off requests, and she was grateful for knowing ahead of time what type of appointments to expect. *"Having had a friend with type 1 who had blazed the trail before me, I was able to be very honest and open with my employer early on to manage their expectation of my time out of the office with all of the appointments. There were so many! Thankfully, a lot of them all in the same building, and frequently we were able to schedule them on the same days. In terms of the hyperintensity, I honestly feel like that is one area of my pregnancy I really knocked out of the park. I don't know what it was, but something inside me just clicked the moment I discovered I was pregnant, and I just knew that taming the diabetes beast was of the utmost importance. To date, the way I managed my diabetes while pregnant remains one of my proudest accomplishments. Thankfully I really wasn't fed any of the myths and misconceptions. I have a really amazing medical team who never once questioned my desire or ability to have a baby."*

During the course of a pregnancy with diabetes, you can't plan for everything. Some things just "happen," and it's not because the parents-to-be didn't work hard enough. Sometimes babies are bigger because they're bigger, not because blood sugars weren't tightly managed during pregnancy. Sometimes birth plans are scrapped because the baby has a different agenda. For me, I was hospitalized with preeclampsia for four weeks before delivering my daughter. I blamed diabetes, and myself, for this issue, but the truth is, it just happened. Same for my scheduled C-section, which was a decision based on the placement of my diabetic retinopathy. I would have preferred avoiding surgery, but my goal was to optimize my health and the health of my daughter, so opting for the C-section was the best choice.

The evening before my C-section, I was a complete wreck. I'd never had any kind of surgery before. I'd never even had an IV. You'd think, after living with type 1 diabetes for more than 23 years, I'd have had my share of hospitalizations, but I was relatively green when it came to anything other than insulin and pump sites.

I was hooked up to an IV line for fluids at about 10 PM on Wednesday, which also served as an emergency glucose drip if I happened to go low overnight. I went to bed that evening with a blood sugar of 109 mg/dL and my baby kicking away inside of me.

And at 5:30 AM on Thursday, I woke up and prepared to meet my daughter. The surgical team at Beth Israel requested that I shower using a special antiseptic soap to prepare my skin for the procedure. After my shower, the nurses came in to connect the insulin drip and disconnect my insulin pump and Dexcom sensor.

At about 6:30 AM, Chris and I went up to the labor and delivery floor of the Beth Israel Deaconess Medical Center.

I was told to dress in the stylish hospital gown and lose all of my undergarments (though I petitioned for—and won rights to wear—my socks). The nurses wheeled me into the triage room, where Chris and I waited for my obstetrician/gynecologist (OB/GYN). While we waited, the nurses carefully monitored my blood sugars with my glucose meter, and I watched as my nerves caused the numbers to rise. Actually, my climbing blood sugars delayed the surgery a little bit, because my medical team wanted me between 80 and 110 mg/dL for the surgery, and I was cresting up toward 160 mg/dL. But once I was holding steady, my OB/GYN came in and said we were ready to administer the spinal block.

The block was starting to take effect, and the team helped me lie on my back and relax my legs. Unfortunately for everyone, the C-section required me to be naked from the sternum down, so basically everyone in the room had a bird's eye view of parts of me I personally hadn't addressed in several weeks. A catheter was set up, a drape was established to block my view of my belly and to keep the lower half of my body sterile, and I was ready for surgery. Ready for my baby to arrive.

My body was completely numb, but I could still feel the pressure of what was taking place down there. It was like having dental work done, where you can't feel the pain but you feel the pressure. I felt them shifting things about inside of me, but it wasn't uncomfortable.

Chris held my hand, and I felt this enormous shifting inside of me. And then the sweetest sound I have ever heard broke through the din of the operating room. The sound reached into my heart and my mind and wrapped around the most vulnerable parts of me and closed tightly, making me feel safe and terrified and excited and ready. It was the sound of my baby's first cry. The child I had been hoping to have for as long as I can remember. My daughter.

"Oh, my baby. It's you. I'm your mommy. I love you." I remember murmuring the same sentences to her, over and over again, marveling at the fact that this tiny baby was just tucked inside of my body, and now she was breathing the same air as me, nestled between her mother and father for the first time in all of our lives.

I looked at Chris, who was staring at his baby with wide, tear-filled eyes. "This is our baby, Chris. She's ours. We did it."

Diabetes is tough. We know that. Diabetes and pregnancy is tough, amplified. But please don't let the stories about what could happen sway you if you are planning to pursue a pregnancy and you have diabetes. The information people share is important, accurate, but can admittedly be overwhelming. Not all pregnancies with diabetes encounter the same kinds of complications—everyone's experiences vary. Just know that information overload comes with any pregnancy, and diabetic ones are no exception. We may get some added bonus worries, but the end result of our pregnancies can be just the same as the pregnancies of non-diabetic women—a healthy baby. It's a lot of hard work, but like they say, it's so, so worth it.

As Karen so eloquently shared, "*Don't be afraid. Do your homework, talk to your doctors, gather a medical team you trust and respect, do the work, but know that the human body is an amazing machine. After nearly twenty years with diabetes, I have a newfound appreciation for my body. What it can do is nothing short of miraculous.*"

Chapter Seven

Parenting with Diabetes

When my daughter was born, I remember staring at her for ages and realizing that all the planning and strategy that had gone into a pregnancy with diabetes were behind me and now I had a baby. An infant, for whom my husband and I were solely responsible. If she cried, it was our job to console her. If she was hungry, it was our job to feed her. And if she smiled, it was our job to feel arrogant and proud, as if we had anything to do with the smile of a two-month-old, when in fact it was most likely gas.

But whatever. We went with it.

Taking diabetes completely out of the equation, the move from "couple" to "couple with a baby" was a tremendous change. My best friend, Lynnae, and her husband became parents for the first time just a few months before Chris and me, so we had a sneak peek at what the transition to parenting might be like. Just after my friend's baby was born, I went over to their house to watch the baby and to give Lynnae a chance to take a nap. I was six and a half months pregnant at the time.

"Here, I can take her for a while and you can go upstairs and nap," I said upon arriving.

"I haven't showered since Tuesday," Lynnae said, running her hands through her blonde hair. "And I don't care."

It was in that moment that I knew life would go bananas once the baby was born. (Thankfully, I quite like bananas.) On some days, diabetes management feels like a full-time job, and I knew that motherhood was going to feel the same way, especially as I adjusted to the change. If my best friend wasn't able to find the time or energy to shower every day, how on earth was I going to balance parenting an infant, recovering from delivery, and staying on top of all the diabetes duties?

I remember the first time I had a very bad low blood sugar, just after we brought the baby home from the hospital. She was tucked into the bassinet, perfectly safe and sound. Only she was wailing with this loud cry, and her bottom lip pouted out at an impossibly steep angle, because she was hungry.

"I'm sorry, baby girl. You have to wait just a few minutes so Mommy can have some juice, okay?"

I was standing at her side, my belly full of grape juice and a blood sugar of 43 mg/dL. My daughter needed to eat. I needed to breast-feed her, but I didn't feel confident picking her up just yet. Of course, she started to cry just as the meter tossed that result at me. A perfect storm of chaos. My hands were too shaky and my brain wasn't 100 percent tuned in to reality, so I felt it was safer to wait instead of picking her up while I still felt dizzy. She was safe and unharmed in her bassinet, but her cries were cutting through me and settling right in like barbed wire around my heart.

"Two more minutes, sweetie. Can you hang on?" I stood by the bassinet and stroked her hair while she cried.

"Why, Mom? Why aren't you picking me up and feeding me? You're right there! I can see you! I can smell you! I hear your voice! Why? Mommy, pick me up!" (Or at least that's what I heard in her cries. I'm sure it was some variation on that theme.)

Within a few more minutes, I felt much better, blood sugar–wise. I felt capable of picking up my daughter and bringing her over to the couch so I could feed her. I kept a jar of glucose tabs on the coffee table while I fed Birdy, and the Dexcom eventually showed some arrows pointing north (it was like receiving a "thumbs up" from my CGM). And we were both fine. Birdy was fed, I was feeling better, and we moved on with our day.

But the guilt of not giving her what she needed, when she needed it, was something to which I needed to adjust. I had to be in good form in order to take good care of my kid. Which meant, in that moment, that tending to a low blood sugar ranked higher than picking up my daughter, in terms of safety. I can't pick her up if I feel shaky. And I can't let the sound of her cries cause me to make decisions that aren't safe. But it was difficult, that struggle between what was best, overall, and what felt necessary, instinct-wise.

Leaving her in the bassinet while I went to drink juice was heartbreaking, because she didn't understand why I wasn't giving her what she needed. I didn't want her to think her mommy was ignoring her. The time will come when she understands how this balance works. She'll grow up knowing that food is sometimes medicine and that her mommy, though madly in love with her, can't do it all at once.

Lindsay Rhoades, T1D and diagnosed at the age of 27, commiserated with me about this. *"I didn't find any balance at first. That's just being honest. For as much as I owned and rocked the hell out of pregnancy, I failed miserably as a new mom with diabetes. My daughter is now two and I still struggle every single day, having to remind myself that my diabetes needs must be a priority, and yes, sometimes even over her wants and needs."*

Yes, a thousand times, yes. This is the challenge of balancing diabetes and parenting—there is no real balance to be struck. The learning curve that comes with being a new parent is so steep and so sleepless that everything feels new, even the diabetes management tasks you could do with your eyes shut. What was once a priority ("Checking my blood sugar first thing every morning! I'm all over it!") becomes something you remember as you're giving your infant their second feeding and you're throwing teeny, spit-up–covered onesies into the washing machine.

Jacquie Wojick agreed. *"I'm still working on this [achieving balance]. I spent a lot of time in post-birth 'screw it all' state, partly because I was so busy taking care of a baby, and partly because I was burned out from the intense control I had during my pregnancy."*

This seems to be a common thread among all the moms I spoke with about pregnancy and subsequent motherhood— the intense diabetes management during pregnancy can lead to patches of diabetes-related burnout. All of that health-focused hard work is in pursuit of achieving a healthy pregnancy, so once the baby is born, your brain might need some breathing room.

I was at Joslin Diabetes Center for an appointment with my endocrinologist a few months after my daughter was born, deep in my own postpartum burnout. We reviewed my blood sugars, of which there were few.

"I'm not checking as much as I'd like to be. Sometimes, I'm taking a fasting number and then not checking again until early afternoon. I'm down to like four times a day. And I'm not going to lie; I wrote these numbers down this morning while sitting in the waiting room. I also made that one up," I said, pointing to a number on the sheet that represented a "before bed" check, but was actually a "before bed" from a completely different day.

She looked at my pathetic logbook and made some notes in her computer system while I purged my diabetic guilt.

"I did great while I was pregnant, didn't I? And then while I was breast-feeding? It seems like, when it mattered for my daughter, I was able to put her first and make my health a priority. But now, I'm in wicked burnout. I don't *care* about a shred of this crap. I don't want to test. I am going through the motions in changing my Dexcom sensor and my pump sites. I'm just ... *pffft* about the whole mess. Is that normal for women after they have a baby, after all the hyperintensive management?"

We talked for a while about how extreme the focus is on diabetes management while pregnant. And how being checked on every week makes for a higher level of accountability and, as a result, a higher level of attention to diabetes. How can things go off the track when you're being monitored so closely?

"It's very common for women to feel burnt out after they have the baby, especially if they are also breast-feeding," my endocrinologist said. "That's more than a year of very intense management. Hopefully checking in with me more often will help get you back on track post-baby?"

This was a step toward balance, or at least restoring some balance to my life. I am not one to take a huge challenge and make a dozen changes, all at once. In order for me to make good health habits that stick, I need to shift things incrementally. The road back from post-pregnancy diabetes burnout and the return to taking responsibility for my diabetes again was a difficult one for me.

Not all new parents experience the burnout that I experienced after becoming a mom. Longtime PWD and friend Melissa Baland Lee felt that motherhood was an easy transition. *"New motherhood came so naturally to me. I don't remember having to balance much of anything. I mean, I kept glucose tabs and juice boxes on my nursing table, but there were so many other things to worry about now. It was nice to be able to shift all of that incessant diabetes attention from the child that cannot be tamed—diabetes—to the child you had for so long longed to hold—your new baby."*

That relief in shifting the focus is something I can identify with, as preparing for and actually being pregnant was a year-long intense focus for me. Motherhood was a more jarring change, being asked to immediately balance baby with "regular life." I didn't find balance, at first, and I don't find it regularly. And this is not something unique to moms with diabetes; dads with diabetes are also making changes to their routine when a child is added to the mix. Diabetes-related tasks and fears can be exacerbated by an expanding family.

"Being a first-time parent with a colicky child, there's honestly very little I clearly remember about the following few months. One of the only ways we could get our daughter to calm down was to walk around the neighborhood with her, and I remember having to do a quick blood sugar check before we headed out to walk around the block. I do remember some middle-of-the-night instances where I had to take

care of my own low blood sugar instead of the crying infant, and that was a hard thing to do. As a parent, you want to do everything you can to make your child happy, but you also have to realize that in order to be able to take care of them, you have to be in working order first," said Harry Thompson, diagnosed with type 1 at the age of eleven and the father of a two-and-a-half-year-old daughter. *"Thankfully my wife was very understanding. And we drank a ton of really strong coffee. I do remember that."*

Harry's diabetes does play into their decision to expand the family, but more because of the residual effects of diabetes. *"I worry that my diabetes will have a major influence on whether or not our daughter has a sibling. Not health-wise, but just from a financial standpoint. While diabetes thankfully isn't quite as expensive as having a child, it's certainly a considerable expense that chips away at the disposable income."*

Worrying about our children developing diabetes can be a pervasive concern in the parenting community, a natural worry considering the disease is something you know so intimately. In my family, most of the decisions we made were born out of the desire for our child to have the best start possible, but diabetes did play an influencing role. When it came to breast-feeding, I decided to do it as her mother, but I worked hard to keep doing it as her mother with diabetes, considering all the research that shows breast-feeding a child can help ward off a type 1 diabetes diagnosis. (But I'm not sure how confident I feel about that, seeing as how I was the only breast-fed child in my family, yet I'm the only one with diabetes. It's a roll of the dice.) My husband and I also decided to delay the introduction of gluten for our daughter until she was 15 months old, based on theories about "leaky gut" serving as an autoimmune catalyst.

George Simmons, diagnosed with type 1 diabetes at the age of 17, is the father of two children who don't have diabetes. "*I have not tested them, at this point, because we all know the symptoms and will check if anything seems odd. But they've both told me that if they were ever diagnosed, they could handle it well because they know so much. My worry is that their kids will have it someday. That almost hurts more than if my own kids developed diabetes. I already feel guilt about even that possibility, like leaving the door open and unknowingly letting a cold burst of air into your warm home.*"

Scott Johnson, diagnosed at age five, is undecided as to testing his own two children. "*On one hand, I am not sure I'd want to know beforehand. I don't want to live life just waiting for the bombshell to drop. But on the other hand, I feel that I am not contributing to the science of diabetes the way I'd like, and I worry that I might miss an important prevention study if either of my kids tested positive for antibodies. It's not an easy issue to wrestle with.*"

Harry was ready to tackle parenthood with his wife, but did have some specific diabetes-related concerns. "*Knowing there's a chance our daughter could someday develop* diabetes, *my wife and I took additional steps that we wouldn't have done otherwise. We decided to bank our daughter's cord blood, admittedly an investment with a potentially low return, but in the event that stem cell research advances to the point where cord-banked blood could actually form the basis of a treatment for a disease, we wanted to prepare for that possibility."*

My husband and I haven't had our daughter formally tested yet, either, for many of the same reasons. I had "the thought" a few times just after my daughter was born. Sometimes it was a very wet diaper that made me furrow my brow. Sometimes she would nurse for longer than usual, and it would give me pause. Even though she seemed (and is) healthy and very strong, I still thought about taking out my meter and pricking her heel myself. And there have been a handful of times when I have checked my daughter's blood sugar, just to put my mind at ease.

Overall, I try to shake the thought off the same way I shake off that thought every time I wonder if my niece or nephew might have dipped into my autoimmune grab bag. I don't allow my brain to go there consistently. It's not denial, but feels more like a protective measure taken by my mind, shielding my psyche from letting fear of something I can't control permeate my daily life. I know what to worry about. I refuse to wait for something to happen that may not ever happen. If her health status were to change, my job is to ensure that her "happy" status doesn't.

Family physician, person with diabetes, and parent of twins, Sean Oser did have to go through the diabetes diagnosis of one of his daughters. Managing her diabetes is a very different journey than managing his own. *"I find it very challenging to manage my own diabetes and my daughter's, often forgetting that they are not the same. I had to start unlearning the 'rules' of diabetes and recasting them as only my own. It was like suddenly learning that gravity doesn't affect everyone the same way, and you feel stupid for not realizing it earlier. On top of that, there was tremendous guilt interwoven with everything, for of course I felt that it was purely my fault that Jessica had developed diabetes; I 'gave it to her.' I've gotten better at shelving the guilt and other emotions to tackle the practical reality of having to manage her diabetes and teach her to do the same, but I'm still learning."*

Guilt, an emotion that seems to hit hard when you are living with diabetes, doesn't make for a good combination alongside the parental guilt that seems to come tucked neatly inside every package of diapers. But diabetes does offer a certain level of perspective, as a parent, and one that offers your child a special perspective all their own.

Sean is concerned that his daughters worry about his diabetes, knowing they both also worry about his daughter's diabetes. *"It's very hard to express and even harder to teach the subtle differences between concern and worry—that one helps you to be prepared while the other can be destructive.*

But my diabetes has definitely helped my children develop a sense of empathy and caring. They understand that disease does not equal disability, and they have seen that something most would mark as 'highly undesirable' can be turned into a source of tremendous strength."

"*My hope is twofold*," said Karen, living with type 1 since she was 15 years old, reflecting on how diabetes touches her daughter's life. "*I hope that she realizes what a gift her healthy body is, and appreciates it and takes care of it, and relishes it. And I also hope that she doesn't need to be held back by any adversity that may come her way. Life isn't always easy, but she'll be strong enough to handle that fact.*"

As an athlete and occasional marathoner, Harry hopes his daughter will eventually understand the need to sometimes put yourself first. "*I know that my diabetes is better controlled when I'm able to exercise regularly, and my body appears to be wired so that I can only commit to an exercise program if I'm training for a specific goal. I end up picking things such as marathons, triathlons, and bike rides that require a considerable amount of training, often cutting into our precious weekend family time.*

"*While I hate spending time away from my family because of training, I hope that our daughter will view the outcome as 'My dad ran a marathon,' rather than 'My dad is sick.' I know it will be a long time before she's able to fully understand diabetes, but I don't get a second chance to give her a first impression of it, and I want her to see that diabetes is not holding me back."*

"*I hope my child learns about self-care,*" offered Melissa. "*My husband and I are from families where self-care was never modeled for us. We saw a lot of self-neglect at the expense of caring for others. Caring for yourself was considered selfish, but I hope that my generation of mothers is teaching their children that we care best for others when we meet our own needs, too. I want my children to watch me count my carbs and go to the doctor and meet others with my condition. I want them to know that we don't hide in the dark with our worries or our obstacles. We take care of ourselves so that we can live life to the fullest.*"

My daughter, if asked what my "job" is, responds, "Your job is to take good care of me." And when I ask her what her job is, she replies, "To take good care of you and Daddy." She understands that part of taking good care of myself means paying attention to diabetes-related things that she barely understands, such as my insulin pump, glucose meter, and the beeps coming from my Dexcom.

"I'm going to draw a picture of Grandpa," she said to me one afternoon.

"Okay, so where do you start?" I asked her.

She put her finger to her lips, pondering. "How about ... a head! With two eyes! And a nose with nostrils. And some cheeks."

Birdy pressed her pen against the paper, painstakingly

drawing a circle for the head, and then two eyes, and a nose. Her attention to detail shows me how much of the world she draws in through her eyes.

"So then ... a neck?" She draws a nice, loooong neck. (Her people sometimes look like kin to giraffes.) "And then some shoulders and a necklace?"

"Does Grandpa wear a necklace?"

"No ... " She thinks again. "He wears a watch. And then ... hmmm ... what else he has on his body?"

"Well, people have lots of the same body parts. Two eyes, two ears, nostrils, teeth, a neck. Look at mommy's body—what do I have that Grandpa also has?"

She surveyed my body closely. "We already has the eyes. And the nose. Oh, knees!!" Pressing the pen to her notebook with satisfaction, some knees were added to her drawing. "But not a Dexcom. You have a Dexcom. You has one but I don't have one. Or Grandpa doesn't have one. You have it."

"True. But what does it do?"

"It goes 'BEEEEEP!' when you need glupose tabs or if you need some insuwin."

"Right. It helps me do my job. Because what's my job?"

"To take good care of me," she says, concentrating hard as she gave Grandpa a second nose.

Chapter Eight

Balancing Diabetes and Love

Diabetes, all on its own, is complicated and unique to each person playing host to it. Add that to the complexity and frailty of romantic relationships and it seems like a powder keg of variability.

So what's the point of this chapter? It's not to make arrogant claims of having figured it out. (*See also: not even close*) It's to make it clear that life with diabetes doesn't equate to a life without love.

My dating life has always included type 1 diabetes, as I was diagnosed just before starting second grade. Actually, my first crush on a boy was also "diagnosed" in second grade. His name was Mike and he let me use his pencil box, which meant we were in love, right? Right. I have clear memories of this first crush, made clearer still by revisiting the journals I kept as a kid.

"Today at school, Mike drew me a picture of a bird," I wrote in my diary, dotting my i's with circles and taping the photo of said bird into the space in the page below. "When he looks at me, I get all fuzzy inside." Was this a mention of a low blood sugar symptom? No way—this was a symptom of puppy love, without any indication of diabetes as part of the thought process. Diabetes, at that time, was new to my life, and it didn't factor into my decision to have a wicked crush on my classmate.

But, further on in my catalog of journals, there is a first mention of diabetes. And it's a bold one: "THERE'S SOMETHING YOU SHOULD KNOW ABOUT ME" the journal entry opens with in all caps, and a list follows. "1. I have type 1 diabetes. 2. I have a really big crush on [insert classmate's name here]." And then the entry rambles on about my then-relevant crush (whose name I can't even bring myself to include, because it still makes me blush that I was so boy crazy in elementary school). But there it is, the first mention of diabetes in the same context as love … or at least near some context of love.

Puppy love is one thing—those first crushes and hormonal surges—but a more grown-up, intense love comes with diabetes as part of the package. It wasn't until I was in my teens that I had a good sense of what the "forever" aspect of diabetes really meant. Diabetes wasn't going anywhere, and if I wanted to fall in love and have happy relationships, I needed to get comfortable with the fact that diabetes came, part and parcel, with all the other aspects of me. For me, that meant disclosing my status as a "person with diabetes" at the very outset of my relationships, almost using that disclosure to aid me in deciding if that person was a potential good fit in my life.

The disclosure, historically, hasn't been a big deal. Boyfriends haven't ever cared. And I like to think that's because I never made it seem like something about which they should worry. They embraced it as part of me because I didn't give them any choice—it was a package deal or no deal. For guys I was dating when I was younger, disclosure came by way of checking my blood sugar in front of them, carefully saying, "I was diagnosed with type 1 diabetes when I was little. Not a big deal, but I need to check my blood sugar and take some insulin before we have dinner." By putting it out there in that casual, "no big deal" sort of way, I felt like I was giving the impression that diabetes was part of what I did, but not the definition of who I was. However, bringing it up early in the courtship (do people even say "courtship" anymore?) highlighted diabetes as something I wasn't ashamed of or hiding. In short, that means that a potential partner needs to be cool with it in order to be cool with me.

My college boyfriend and I were still dating when I transitioned from injecting insulin to using an insulin pump. I had been on injections for almost two decades before deciding to make the leap to pumping insulin, and the main reason I decided to use an insulin pump was because I was interested in having children. Not at that moment, but children were part of the future I was hoping to have, and I knew that the better I could manage my blood sugars, the better chance I'd have of a healthy pregnancy. It was kind of a heavy thought process for a dating relationship that danced on the delicate precipice of having, or not having, children, since my boyfriend at the time was vehemently against parenthood as part of his own future.

"But I want to do this. And I know that means, eventually, I'll do this without you. But this is about me, and I know I'll regret not trying." The decision to pump insulin was my first, early step toward motherhood, and with that step came the end of a very meaningful, but ultimately very mismatched, relationship.

Even still, my college boyfriend went through the transition to pumping as though he were in it for the long haul. "Even if we aren't together, years from now, I want you to be as healthy as you can be." My first few weeks of pump training, and then pump implementation, were with my boyfriend at my side, emotionally supporting my decision and even opting to wear his own "insulin pump"—a piece of yarn connected to his abdomen by way of a Band-Aid, snaking out to meet a key fob he kept in his pocket to simulate the weight and presence of an insulin pump.

That relationship melted away once my mission of future motherhood was established, but ultimately left me with the feeling that diabetes was not something that dictated who loved me, or whom I loved, and gave me the confidence that my disease did not dictate whom I dated. Armed with this confidence and taking huge strides in owning my diabetes, I met my now-husband, Chris.

Our relationship from the start was one rooted in affection and attraction, with diabetes as a backburner issue. Chris wasn't a diabetes expert, by any stretch, but he did have a basic knowledge of the disease when we first met. "*I had really limited exposure to type 1 diabetes, but I knew that type 2 existed. I knew that certain foods drove up blood sugar levels, but that information was all tied to previous exposure to type 2 diabetes,*" he said. "*I fell into the category of people who mistakenly stereotyped diabetes as belonging solely to people who were overweight and old.*"

"But you've learned a lot since," I said, reminding him of the day we first met, when I was at our shared office and he was visiting for the week. He noticed my insulin pump, which was clipped to the waistband of my pants.

"*I have. Before you, everything I knew about type 1 diabetes was tied to a girl one of my friends used to date. She wore a pump, just like the one you had on, and it didn't seem like a big deal. She seemed fine—healthy and fit. The only weird thing I ever noticed was, one Halloween, I witnessed an argument between her and my friend. She was having a low blood sugar reaction, and during the course of the argument, she threw a pumpkin. So that was it for me—*

type 1 diabetes involved wearing pumps and throwing pump-kins." He smiled. *"I've come a very long way since then, but I really didn't have a clue. Knowing more wouldn't have changed my thoughts or feelings, but at the time, you wearing a plastic device all the time didn't faze me in the slightest."*

There is no one "right" way to disclose diabetes to a potential romantic partner. People's preferences vary from person to person, and couple to couple. In my life, quick disclosure was my way of "ripping the Band-Aid off quickly," because once that information tidbit was out, I felt comfortable and ready to leave it as much behind as possible, until it warranted further discussion. I spoke with Karen Graffeo and her husband, Pete, about how they handled Karen's diabetes in the early stages, as their discussions varied greatly from mine.

"When we first got together, I was still at a stage in my life when I hated for anyone to know I had diabetes. For the first few months, I hid it from Pete, doing my injections in the bathroom and skipping blood sugar checks. I finally told him on our first weekend away together. We were on a beach with some wine and cheese, watching the sunset, and I took a deep breath and told him I had something important to tell him. Pete let me know he was willing to learn about diabetes right from the outset, but at that point, I mostly handled things myself. And as we moved along, it was something we discussed in bits. But now, after almost 14 years together, Pete knows as much about diabetes as I do. The closer we

became, the more diabetes wove itself into our life together."

Similarly, my husband and I practiced the "learn as we get to know one another" method of handling diabetes. He didn't realize how serious diabetes was, or could be, until he saw me have my first serious low blood sugar.

("You're really going to write about this?" he asked me, as I was interviewing him for this chapter. "I guess. It was kind of a significant moment," I replied. So here we go.)

"*Okay, then. So, admittedly, I jokingly tried to take credit for that low blood sugar after the fact, especially since I had zero idea what a low actually looked like, or how it affected you. But it was right after we had sex for the first time, and ...*"

"Can you say, 'first time we were intimate,'" I interrupted.

"*Fine. It was the first time we were intimate and right afterwards, we were all sweaty and whatnot ... actually, you were all sweaty. And you looked confused. And then you said you needed juice, right away. So I ran to get juice, right away.*"

"This is the awkward part."

"*Exactly. No one wants to talk about post-sex running around. But you needed juice, and I had to get it for you. It seemed so serious, and you looked panicked. And, after you had the juice and your blood sugar started to come up, we talked about it. But waiting for you to 'come back' felt like a very long couple of minutes.*"

In retrospect, I wish I had talked with Chris about the lag

time between treating a low blood sugar and when I'd start speaking coherently again. The curve for "learning about" and "teaching about" was steep on both sides. I always wondered what it would be like to date another person with diabetes, to have that unique and intimate understanding that almost happens without explanation.

Dayle Kern and Christopher Snider dated for three years, and both are living with type 1 diabetes, so they understand firsthand what it's like to live with diabetes and also care for someone else's diabetes. But disclosure wasn't an issue for either of them, as a job e-mail thread disclosed for them.

"Dayle found me through my diabetes blog. She was tasked with a blogger outreach event for the American Diabetes Association. In Dayle's initial e-mail to me, she mentioned her own issues with dawn phenomenon, so from that opening correspondence, our respective diabetes was out in the open. I guess I was lucky in that I never had to hide anything or build up the strength to talk about it, early on. But I will admit that I was too embarrassed to bring my meter to our first get together. As if I had something to hide from her. Since then, I've become more comfortable with my diabetes around her, and in general. I think being close to someone with an intimate familiarity helped me mature with respect to how I view my diabetes in public situations."

Seeing diabetes reflected, in tandem, in your relationship is a whole new level of understanding. Christopher talks about watching Dayle coming up after her own low blood sugar, and the helplessness that came in waves.

"*Diabetes is quite crafty in its ability to break a person down. But that kind of helplessness is when it's my blood glucose. I think I feel even more helpless when that low blood glucose registers on her meter. I can get a Capri Sun or glucose tabs for her, no problem, but then the waiting game starts. I hate waiting for the correction to kick in. I hate that I can't do any more than what I've already done. I want to move mountains but have to settle for twiddling my thumbs. I literally know exactly what she's going through, but I can't settle on the fact that I've done all that I can. I'm glad I can be around to help out, but seeing what diabetes can do to her is a thousand times worse than whatever it can do or has done to me. If I could take on twice the diabetes so she didn't have to deal with any of this, I would.*"

Even though he doesn't experience the sensation himself, my husband has seen his share of hypoglycemic events. "*There's this detachment that comes over you, when your blood sugar is really low. Your eyes kind of gloss over, and you don't seem to be focusing on anything, more looking through whatever is in front of you. If it's a low in the middle of the night, while we're sleeping, you wake me up and ask for juice or glucose tabs, but your voice has this disembodied, ethereal quality to it. It's like you're possessed. I don't worry as much, now that you wear a CGM and we hear the alarms when you're low on the overnight. But before you were on the Dexcom, I would wake at night and my first instinct would* be to touch your forehead, to see if you were sweating."

With any relationship, I'd imagine there is fear about what the future might be like, or how everyone's health may fare in his or her lifetime together. With diabetes, some of that fear already has a name and has been faced with regularity, in the shape of severe blood sugar excursions and the threat of diabetes-related complications in the future.

"*I don't get worked up about things until there's something to be worked up about*," offered my husband, talking about what our own future may include. "*I've seen some really bad low blood sugars, and I've seen you scared. Seeing you scared made me scared, but it felt temporary. Perception is my reality—you seem young, vibrant, smiling, out there exercising and working and taking care of our daughter. I guess proof of my lack of worry is that we have these massive, blow-out fights sometimes—if I was so worried about diabetes making you fragile, wouldn't we be walking on eggshells? No, we fight and make up and live like any other couple. I don't think about all these things that 'might happen.' You and I work hard to make sure we're both healthy, and if anything changes, we'll deal with that together.*"

Karen and Pete shared a similar sentiment. "*In the present, diabetes makes me try harder to take care of myself because I want to be around as long as I can and be as healthy as I can be for Pete,*" Karen said. "*As for the future, I often worry about dying young and leaving him alone.*"

Pete remained steadfast in the simplicity of his love for his wife. *"I don't think it really has much of an impact on the present. I love her, diabetes and all. My same feelings go for the future."*

But what if you haven't found your significant other yet? What if diabetes is part of what holds you back in relationships? Does diabetes play a part in relationship anxiety?

Briley Boisvert, in her early twenties and in the dating pool, finds disclosure to be a little awkward and somewhat intimidating. *"Diabetes and dating are intimidating because I know that it's technically not a big deal, but I get nervous and flustered on dates, making explaining diabetes as no big deal more difficult. In the beginning it's just about getting to know each other. Do I like this person? Do we like to do some of the same things? Do we laugh at the same things? Diabetes is going to come up in bits and pieces. Like if I take baby food out of my purse on a date, I'm going to need to explain why, and hopefully he won't think I'm too crazy. And when I bolus for drinks or food or check my BG before getting in my car to go home; those will need explaining, too. I think that explaining something as all-encompassing as diabetes is hard, so to have him have a basic understanding before that conversation happens is important. When the big diabetes conversation is going to seem a little less intimidating, that is when I'm most comfortable having it."*

But she worries. *"I mostly worry about the moment when a low will come and interfere. I worry about the nights that*

I need five juice boxes to wake up in the morning and how weak it makes me feel. I worry that a sweat-producing low will affect me right before a first date, making me go from 'pretty' to 'pretty messed-up.' I worry about the lows that make me scared to be alone, and make me want to call him, even though I've only explained diabetes as 'no big deal.' And I worry about the highs that make me a bitch. When will I snap and will I have explained it before I do? Will he accept my unintentional and sporadic weakness? Will he understand that being surrounded by people with diabetes is really important because it's the only time when I'm with people who understand the part of me I didn't get to choose? I've got a whole basket of crazy to bring along with me that can't be dropped off anywhere, no matter how hard I try."

Briley is not alone in her concerns, but there is a balance to be found between making diabetes part of the relationship and then making it the focus of the relationship. *"I think that the most important thing about diabetes and relationships is that diabetes is just a piece of who I am. Yes it will come in and steal the show every once in a while, but what's more important is what the actual show was. There are going to be times when I'm going to complain and I won't be able to focus on anything else. There are going to be times when I want to snap your head off, because it's not like I can yell at my pancreas. Please love me just the same. Love me for me, and accept that diabetes will interrupt sometimes."*

Christopher Snider does his best to allay Briley's concerns.

"Diabetes doesn't really matter when it comes to love. It's one of the least important factors in how I am as a partner in my relationships. But it does matter for people who are the only person with diabetes in the relationship, because in that situation, you've gained a new advocate. It's nice to expand that kind of support."

A malfunctioning pancreas doesn't mean you aren't capable of giving or receiving tremendous love. There's nothing sweeter (sorry for another bad pun) than accepting yourself, and if you accept yourself, the chances of a potential partner accepting you are infinitely higher.

Chapter Nine

Walking the Blood Sugar Tightrope

After living with type 1 diabetes for almost three decades, I've come to realize that nothing works more efficiently and effectively than a properly functioning pancreas. All my insulin pumps and continuous glucose monitors and exercise can only take me so far. That's the reality of life with diabetes: it's not a perfect science, and perfect diabetes management isn't an achievable goal. (Not to mention, it's a constantly moving target.)

Knowing that perfection isn't possible makes dealing with the day-to-day of diabetes a little easier. When I check, I know that my blood sugar isn't going to be between 80 to 110 mg/dL every time. Seeing those numbers is a cause for celebration, but seeing numbers that aren't within that range isn't a reason to hang my head. Letting those kinds of discouraging thoughts enter my head isn't healthy. I need to find ways to stop myself from assigning emotional worth to my blood sugars. Instead, I need to see them as what they are—information.

I'm not sure when it started, but while I was growing up blood sugars were either "good" or "bad." I don't fault my parents or my endocrinologist, but more the perception that we had so many tools to manage diabetes, so of course we should be able to hit all the suggested marks! Also, "good" is easy to reward by way of Barbie Dolls and being allowed to stay up late, but each "good" comes with a guilt-inducing "bad" counterpart.

I have a hard time with some of the adjectives assigned to blood sugar results. When that 52 mg/dL result grins up at me from my meter, I have to beat back the phrases that jump into my head. "Bad number!" "What did I do?" "Wrong!" "Scary!" Same for the 342 mg/dL that comes with the same knee-jerk reaction of blame and shame.

It's a psychological war zone, attaching these types of emotions to blood sugar management. Walking the tightrope in pursuit of in-range numbers is difficult enough, with all the variables, but positioning the rope over a nest of emotions-in-the-shape-of-alligators makes it that much harder.

"The emotions surrounding the numbers would be fine if they only served to motivate us to take better care of ourselves. But instead, they can make us feel disappointed, ashamed, or angry. They slowly break us down and chip away at our confidence in dealing with diabetes," says

Dr. Shara Bialo, pediatric endocrinologist and a 20-year veteran of type 1 diabetes. *"Every blood glucose check is interpreted as a mini-test of our abilities, and no one wants to see a failing grade, myself included.*

"Both patients and physicians gather data in an effort to better control diabetes. Data and numbers are scientific and it is only natural to look at diabetes like a concrete math problem. If you add the same elements together, you should get the same result each time. Diabetes, though full of numbers, rarely gives you the same result day after day. This is immensely frustrating for me as a patient in dealing with my own diabetes, and can be even more frustrating when I am trying to decode a patient's glucose records in order to help them."

Blood sugar management is truly like walking a tightrope, needing to carefully balance the numbers, and the emotions tied to those numbers. I've started removing the words *good* and *bad* from my blood sugar vocabulary. They've been replaced with *in range* and *out of range*, or *high* and *low*. Something as simple as redefining the adjectives associated with each meter reading makes the result easier to learn from and to move past. These numbers don't define me, and they don't define my life. What they represent is information about my diabetes control, and they give me a point from which to start again. Low, high, or right in range, I need to stop fearing the result and instead start learning from it.

Dr. Jill Weissberg-Benchell, licensed clinical psychologist

and certified diabetes educator, feels strongly about the need to know your numbers. *"I don't care what your blood sugar number actually is. I honestly don't care. I don't care if your meter reads 'Hi,' and I don't care if it reads '39.' What I care about is that you check, and when you get a number that is not in your target range, you know what to do, and then you do it."*

Sometimes getting people with diabetes to check in the first place can be a hurdle. I'll attest to this—if I know my blood sugar is high, there are times when I don't want to prick my finger and see confirmation of that high. That number, as Shara mentioned, contributes to feelings of having failed. And when I'm already feeling crummy as a result of the high blood sugar, the failure feeling adds insult to injury.

I spoke about that avoidance concept with Jill, and she confirmed that she hears that sort of sentiment from her patients all the time. *"Patients tell me, 'I know my number is high, and therefore I don't want confirmation, because knowing that number means I'm a screw up.' But some people are socialized in that way to feel that 'numbers are everything' and that numbers are report cards for being a good or bad human being."*

Sean Oser has been living with type 1 diabetes for 24 years and works as a family physician. One of his twin daughters was diagnosed with type 1 diabetes when she was seven, making him both a PWD, the parent of a PWD, and a health-care professional. The guy wears a lot of hats, and it can be challenging to not see diabetes through all of those different perspectives. *"Regarding 'good' and 'bad' in general, I don't recall any specific direction about this when I was diagnosed with type 1 diabetes at 17 years old. However, when my daughter was diagnosed with diabetes 20 years later, but 10 years younger than I was at my diagnosis, her team was emphatic about one of the things I remember most clearly about the blurry day of her diagnosis: 'There are no good or bad blood sugars; every result is just a number, and it tells us what to do next.' This was incredibly helpful and supportive at the time, and it comes in very handy now, a few years later, during those times when she's having a diabetes meltdown. I've told patients of mine the same thing when I've sensed they might have fragile feelings about 'their control' and need me to help reduce the load they carry. But my own blood sugars are definitely either good or bad. The emotional toll of dealing with so much personal data must be great, but I think we adapt to it quickly and often don't realize—or at least we underestimate—the constant judgments we make about our numbers, and by extension about ourselves."*

So how do we fix this head game that diabetes plays with our emotions? *"Prevention is best,"* said Jill. *"If you can't prevent, then the next best thing is to begin to challenge those thoughts that are maladaptive or inaccurate ... because they aren't getting you anywhere. Become your own best litigator! There are all kinds of methods of treating patients that were once accepted as 'medical knowledge,' that we're now, like,*

'How the hell did we ever think that way?'

How do you move past these thoughts of failure? Acknowledge the imperfect nature of insulin. And the imperfect accuracy of these blood sugar meters. Yet we base our judgments of ourselves on these imperfect measurements? There are no data to support the belief that out-of-range numbers are a result of your own personal failure as a human being. An unknown number is where the danger occurs. You can't fix a number you don't know."

Shara feels that addressing the physical needs of diabetes can't be done without simultaneously tending to the psychosocial needs. "I feel the emotional needs and the physical needs of diabetes are so intricately woven together that it is impossible to separate them. The physical aspect of diabetes affects emotion. If I do not count carbohydrates carefully and end up hyperglycemic, it physically makes me feel like molasses and weighs me down mentally. When I have had a day full of lows, I find my mood is more fragile than usual. When life gets emotionally stressful, my blood sugar skyrockets or plummets depending on the situation. It seems as though everything affects diabetes, and diabetes affects everything.

"That is why it is so important to not ignore emotional well-being, and I believe it should be ranked above all else," Shara continued. "You cannot have a healthy body without a healthy mind, because the mind runs the show. If it were up to me, personal and family-centered counseling would *be mandatory at diagnosis and every few years thereafter. Everyone would get a psychological checkup, the same way we get physical exams each year. I have taken advantage of counseling services in the past for the sole purpose of managing the swirl of emotions surrounding my life with diabetes. I always make sure to pay the most attention to the emotional side. The physical aspect will then follow suit."*

As a person who has had diabetes for many decades, I have found once I'm in a good routine of checking and paying attention, I'm good, but it's tough to stick with that program for months on end without a few hiccups of diabetes burnout. Burnout is a tricky little monster because it can sneak up on you and then you're in it, without realizing how or when you ended up in that mental state. Feeling guilty and ashamed of certain results to the point where you don't react to and act upon the numbers is a tough spot to be in, but understanding those numbers and how to fix them empowers us.

Jill talked with me about how burnout can lead to depression, and how, with practice, you can make your emotional responses actually work in your favor. *"We know that depression, in part, comes from a sense of learned helplessness. 'When I am not able to achieve my goals, despite putting energy in, I feel helpless. When I feel helpless, I feel sad and give up.' This way of thinking leads to feelings of depression. In a diabetes sense, the thoughts can be, 'I can't get my numbers right. I work hard. No matter what I do, and the outcome is not what I expected or hoped for.' Do you beat yourself up about that, or do you take stock and assess?*

"You have an event—a blood sugar number, let's say—and you have thoughts about why did this happen? And you also have thoughts about the consequences of it having happened, consequences like, 'My parents will hate me, my doctors will yell at me,' et cetera. Your beliefs about why this happened and what happens next drive your emotional responses and your actions. The challenge is that, if your beliefs are not accurate, then you're feeling like a mess for no reason, and then the choices you make are not adaptive because they are based on inaccurate data. Have your feelings, but make them take you somewhere useful. With practice—and a LOT of it—you will stop and think about this, and that will give you more of a sense that you get to choose. This puts the power back to the person, takes away the helplessness."

Shara agreed. *"Many of our patients let diabetes fall by the wayside and then have a really hard time successfully taking it on again. I went through my own very long period of poor control and was only able to break it thanks to some persistently patient doctors and CDEs. I apply what I learned from my experience to my patients going through the same. The bottom line is to avoid taking on too many goals at the same time.*

"For example, some patients only check their blood glucose once a day—or way less. As their physician, if I demand that they start checking six times a day, as well as

to ensure insulin is administered with each snack (not just meals), and to log everything, and to exercise at least three times a week, it will feel like an impossibly tall order. So I start small. I focus on forming mini-goals and offer several from which to choose, such as checking two times a day instead of one time or taking insulin with snacks, but not both. People often leave the doctor's office with 15 promises to do better, but that becomes overwhelming and ultimately unsustainable. Then we find that nothing changes in between visits. Instead, we can decide on only one or two goals together. Once the goal is met and conquered, we can add another."

Jill aims to make goals relevant to her patients, to help amp up their motivation. "I work with some teenagers who are running blood sugar averages in the 300s, sometimes 400s, and I need to find a way to make it matter to them. But they don't want to hear about complications and things later down the road—they need something that's relevant to them, where they are now. So I will approach them and ask if they wake up at night to go pee. Of course they do. And of course they hate it. They're teenagers, so they all want to sleep 15 hours. I am now talking to them about an experience that matters to them. So they say, 'Yeah, I hate waking up in the middle of the night to go pee.' This opens the door for me to say, 'Are you willing to work with me about strategies to make that stop?' And there it is: something relevant to them, right in that moment. It's a goal *they want to achieve. It's meaningful, right now."*

So once you're in a routine that is a good one, you should be good to go, right? Is it enough to be ticking off items on the to-do list, or do we, as people with diabetes, need to constantly re-educate ourselves regarding the best course of action?

Sean drives home the point that we need to do more than go through the motions. *"As the years go by and we become accustomed to life with diabetes to the point that it just seems like a normal part of life, we risk letting diabetes run on autopilot. Injections may be taken faithfully, sliding scales may be followed reliably, but if there is no ongoing active thinking, we have autopilot. We should continue to hone our carb counting skills, analyze our numbers rather than simply record them, and educate ourselves about advances in management and not let autopilot assume control."*

But is there a balance between autopilot and burnout? *"I have no idea how I balance the emotional and physical needs of diabetes. I'm not even sure I do,"* admitted Sean. *"The emotional balance is harder. Exercise helps a lot with emotional balance in general for me, including the emotional demands of diabetes, but it stretches far beyond that. I always feel better emotionally after a demanding workout. Reminding myself to set a better example for my daughter is an emotional burden, but also a motivator, and it thereby helps me maintain some emotional balance as well. The love and support of my family are essential and greatly appreciated. Those*

things are necessary but not sufficient, though, without per-
sonal connections with other PWDs, which is a key to my
emotional balance. Before I had any such connections, exer-
cise, my family, and my role model to daughter tightrope
walk were not enough, and I wavered between autopilot and
burnout, neither of which was healthy. I'm in a much better
and much healthier place now, which I wouldn't be without
my diabetes friends."

Diabetes isn't just a physiological disease. It's an emotional one, too. It's not just a question of blood sugar levels and in-sulin supplementation. It's about managing the emotions that come as part of life with a chronic illness. It's about the guilt of complications. The pressure to control an uncontrollable disease. The hope that tomorrow will come without incident. I feel that the emotional aspects of diabetes need to be at-tended to with the same care and diligence as an A1C level, because at the end of the day, happiness is the goal.

Like Sean and many others, I have the best diabetes man-agement moments when I feel both emotionally and physi-cally equipped to do what needs to be done. If my head is in a good place, I'm more apt to check my blood sugar and react to those numbers in a healthy way. It wasn't until I had access to other people living with diabetes, by connecting through the Internet and by way of diabetes conferences, that I was able to peel off some of the adjectives I had previously stuck to my blood sugar results and to see them simply as what they are—data points, not measures of my self-worth.

Chapter Ten

Fitting Diabetes Devices into Daily Life

When I was diagnosed with diabetes, there weren't a lot of options for treatment. I needed insulin immediately, so when I was seven, I started taking injections. At first, I was only taking two shots a day, but as the years progressed, insulin changed and my treatment goals shifted. I needed to take more injections in order to achieve the best results. When I was about 23 years old, I realized I was taking upward of nine injections a day: a morning Lantus dose (long-acting), three pre-meal boluses, two or three pre-snack boluses, and an evening Lantus dose. Add in a correction bolus here and there and I was poking holes into my skin every time I even thought about food.

I wanted to try out an insulin pump. I was itching for something that gave me tighter control opportunities without making my skin feel excessively porous. And even though I was in my early twenties and had yet to meet my now-husband, I was always thinking about that baby I knew I wanted to have someday. An A1C closer to that "healthy baby" range was my goal, and I knew a pump would help me get there.

But it's an external device! A *thing* hanging from a tube on my body. Was I ready for an external symptom of diabetes? Was I willing to give up true nudity in favor of cyborg badassery?

My pump arrived via special overnight delivery. On a Saturday, no less. The room shrank as the box sat unopened.

I made myself a cup of tea and sat down on the floor. Peeled back the packing tape. The flaps sprang open and a few stray foam peanuts flung themselves onto the floor, falling victim to the big paws of my calico cat. Reaching into the box, I foraged around until I found the green, white, and blue box inside. "Medtronic MiniMed. Paradigm 512."

It looked like a pager. Slightly bigger, maybe, weighing in at just a few ounces. Smokey gray in color and almost transparent, I could see all the gears and wires inside.

Sipping my tea, I clipped it to the top of my shorts and stood up, to test it out. I felt unbalanced, as though I would tip to one side if an aggressive breeze blew through. Leaving it attached, I jumped up and down. Nothing happened. I sat on the couch to see if I would feel its presence. I walked over to the window and looked out onto the deck, hearing the soft clink of the pump as it touched against the window sill.

The box of infusion sets was decidedly dodgier. Twenty-three inches of snaky, thin white tubing. The round white patch of gauze with the bright blue lid on it. A 6 mm cannula.

Prying open the infusion set packaging, I touched the tip of the needle with my finger. It was hollow and very sharp. I lifted up my shirt and exposed my stomach, daring myself to press the needle tip against my skin. It stung a small bit, but no more than a syringe.

I was used to syringes, though. I'd used them many times a day for more than 17 years. Was I ready for this? This change? This whole new regimen?

I pressed the needle hard against my stomach, watching as my skin resisted, then that sliding *pop* of compliance as the needle slid in. I pulled out the blue cap and inspected the infusion set in my stomach for the first time. It looked like the cap on children's Tylenol. Like a tiny little Superdome on my abdomen.

Standing in front of the full-length mirror in my bathroom, it was bright white against my skin. I pulled my shirt tight over it and saw its outline against the fabric. It didn't hurt. It wasn't big. It could go unnoticed. My body still looked the same. I was still the same.

To be honest, I was completely creeped out at first. But why? This small thing, clipped to my belt and the cannula under my skin, was going to help me achieve better control. It was going to assist me in lowering my otherwise-plateaued A1C. The pump was going to afford me the freedom of sleeping late, conquering the dawn phenomenon, and bolusing minute increments.

I felt different, though. This pump was the first external sign of my diabetes. And that, after 17 years of quiet injections and subtle finger pricks, stirred up the oddest combination of pride and fear. I had done this for so long the only way I knew how. This new method was daunting. I had no idea that my A1C would drop within three months. Or that I would sleep late on a Saturday and not end up hypoglycemic. Or that I would feel strikingly healthier and confidently safer ten years later.

I felt so changed, like it was an extra arm hanging from my body and not a small medical device, but at the same time, it was both startling and comforting to look in the mirror and still see me.

I realized that the device I had just installed on my body, unlike the disease itself, was not permanent. The only thing that was permanent, pending a cure for diabetes, is my need for synthetic insulin. I can choose to deliver it, insurance gods willing, by whatever method works best for me. For almost ten years now, I've been delivering my insulin via insulin pump, sending insulin from a cartridge lodged in a pager-like device, shooting down a plastic tube and into a cannula that's inserted underneath my skin. It's the method that allows me the flexibility in food choices, sleep schedules, and basal rates that I want to have.

But. (And this is a big but.) It's removable. A tattoo would be more permanent than this device. On the days when my pump doesn't quite fit into my clothing choices, or when I'm going through patches of diabetes burnout, I can opt to remove the pump for a few days/weeks and return to the regimen of multiple daily injections.

When I started pumping, I felt that, for the first time in my life, I had treatment options. And it felt good to have those options. Feeling empowered by the newness of options, I felt confident enough to try a continuous glucose monitor (CGM), sticking my first Dexcom sensor to my skin and reveling in the fact that it gave me streaming video of my blood sugar results, when I had had access only to snapshots for the last 20 years.

With these external devices, however, comes the need to integrate them into our daily lives. It's not like we spend the day at home, wearing clothes that cater to our diabetes, putting ourselves only in situations that play nice with diabetes. Life with diabetes means "life," and these technology bits and pieces needed to find a way to blend in.

"I can't stand having things attached to my belt, so I always keep my pump in my left front pocket," offered Harry Thompson, diagnosed with type 1 diabetes when he was 11 years old. *"To avoid having tubing coming out of my pocket and under my shirt, I cut a little hole in the inside of the pocket to snake the tubing inside my pants and up to the abdomen/back/wherever my infusion set happens to be. When I first started doing this, I would hem the fabric*

around this hole so that it looked a lot like a button hole and wouldn't easily unravel. Now I don't bother and I just cut the hole. Sure, I may lose a dime or two through the tubing hole every now and then, but that's quite literally a small price to pay for comfort."

Hiding a diabetes device during the course of a regular day is one thing, but what about special occasions? Like your wedding day, perhaps? When Chris and I were married in May of 2008, wearing the insulin pump was the easiest and least intrusive way for me to take my insulin, and I wasn't about to go off the pump just for the sake of fashion. (Besides, my wedding day was a day when I wanted to worry least about diabetes, so I wanted to stick with what was working for me.) My solution? Design a pocket to hold my insulin pump, hidden in my wedding dress. I spoke with the seamstress at my bridal shop, and she and I designed a pocket in my wedding dress that left the pump accessible, yet hidden.

The pocket itself was underneath the main fabric of the dress, attached to the petticoat. It was sized to be about half an inch bigger than my insulin pump, leaving room for my hands to reach in and access the pump. We stuck a safety pin to the top of the pocket so that, when I reached in, I could feel around quickly for the pin and know exactly where the top of the pocket was located. This made pump retrieval and replacement very easy. The tubing itself went from the top of the pump, through a hole cut into the petticoat, and attached to the infusion site on my right thigh. I had to plan ahead of time where my infusion set would be located so the pocket could be properly situated.

And during the entire course of my wedding, no one had any clue that I was wearing my insulin pump in my wedding dress. Even my friends who knew about it couldn't find it unless I pointed it out. I felt empowered and like a secret agent ... only the bridal version.

Karen Hoffman, diagnosed with type 1 at age 15, finds herself seeking a wardrobe that does the work for her when it comes to diabetes devices. *"As the years have progressed, I find myself buying clothes that accommodate my gear rather than the other way around, though I do have one of those spandex thigh holster things that has served me well for most dresses. My big MacGyver moment was for a bridesmaid dress I had to wear for a formal wedding. I thought hiking my floor-length gown up anytime I needed to access my MiniMed pump was a little, ahem, uncouth, so the seamstress made a pocket when she was doing all the other usual alterations. Worked like a charm!"*

But the best-laid plans don't always work out according to specifications. *"When my husband and I got married a few years ago, I had to figure out how the dress could accommodate the insulin pump I was wearing,"* said Kim Vlasnik, who has been living with type 1 diabetes since she was six. *"I had no idea that some women opted to have a tailor add an interior pocket to their dress. I thought I was stuck with my usual methods of hiding it in my underwear somewhere. I thought I had found a place on my hip (and beneath my Spanx) that would work, but as the warm June day wore on, I was proven wrong. On the drive to our reception dinner, the pump died! Lesson learned—even insulin pumps need breathing room."*

Similar to Kim, Christopher Angell (diagnosed at age 30) once fried his continuous glucose monitoring receiver. *"I tried taking my Dexcom Seven Plus surfing once, and the waterproof case I bought leaked a little … and the salt water fried it. That was an expensive experiment that kept me from trying again until recently."* But once he figured out how to make it work, it was worth it. *"I took my G4 [Dexcom] surfing last week for the first time and it worked out fine. I didn't ever look at the actual screen, but I could feel the vibrations, so I would have known if I was dropping, and for the first time, I had a graph of my blood glucose while I was surfing."*

Part of the power of these devices comes in their ability to make things like exercising easier. As Chris mentioned with his experiences surfing, knowing the trends of your blood sugars while exercising can be a powerful safety net. And Harry finds the insulin pump to be beneficial for him when it comes to running. *"When I was on multiple daily injections (MDI), I became really frustrated with the fact that I couldn't just solve one problem without affecting everything else during the day. If I took enough long-acting insulin to fight off my dawn phenomenon highs, I'd be low the rest of the day. If I reduced my long-acting dose because of an athletic event, I'd be okay during the event but high before and after. I really just got sick of making compromises, and I've found that the pump has given me the freedom to not have to plan my life 24 hours in advance."*

But another aspect of living with a diabetes device—or several—is that it's not just the physical device you're managing, but the psychosocial implications, as well. I felt that when I put on the insulin pump for the very first time, and again with the CGM. These seemingly small, innocuous bits of technology look so tiny in the boxes they come packaged in, but pressed against, and into, my skin? It's a different story. For years, my body didn't look "diabetic," and undressed, I looked the same as anyone without diabetes. Working diabetes devices into my life was a tough transition for me, and while I'm grateful for the benefit of these bionic bits, there are still days when the data are too much to mentally process. I sometimes miss having a physical canvas untouched by technology. For the most part, wearing a pump and a CGM isn't something I feel self-conscious about, but being honest, there are days when I want to rip them both off and throw them across the room in pursuit of feeling truly naked. I dance between the edges of "fine with it," "empowered by it," and "over it." I don't like having these artificial bits and pieces stuck to me all the time, but I try to keep tabs on the bigger picture, which is my overall health. Sounds cheesy, but it's the truth.

Blair Ryan was diagnosed with type 1 diabetes at the age of 14 and used an insulin pump for 12 years before returning to MDI. Initially she resisted using a CGM out of fear that the potential data overload provided by diabetes devices would be overwhelming, confident that she took care to keep what can be tracked in mind. *"At any moment, my blood sugar is the result of an accumulation of physiological factors and diabetes management decisions. Most often, I am aware of why my blood sugar is what it is because of 13 years of life with diabetes and the trials and errors that come with time. I would know this information without the devices I use. I don't need a CGM to tell me that I'm 320 mg/dL; I can tell by the way I have to pee, and that feeling is much more revealing of my health than the number on the screen."* Blair started using a CGM in 2012 for convenience during exercise, and intends to continue using it indefinitely. *"Just like there are times to ignore the data and live your life, there are times to use the data to force you to be realistic and make timely decisions. There is nothing you can do to take back a blood sugar result, but you will have the data and experience that led to it in your toolbox for the future."*

I realize it can sound a little blasphemous to say "ignore the data," especially when we, as a community, fight for access to this technology through insurance coverage and company policies. But it is important to turn off the diabetes noise sometimes, because if you're not in a good mental place to deal with it, it can become something that contributes to unsettled emotional health. The data are only good if you are in a position to do something useful with them.

Kim agreed. "*I have been known to shut down my CGM receiver when it's blatantly lying, or when it hasn't quite calibrated correctly, or when I'm trying to sleep because sometimes I'm just like, 'Would you just stop beeping already!?'*"

The same goes for me. There are days when, after dealing with itchy rashes that are a reaction to adhesive tape, and doorknobs tugging hard on pump tubing, and just feeling a little excessively robotic over the last few weeks, I wanted to disconnect and decompress for a few days. What I like most is having options. I prefer the pump for long-term use, but I like that I can take it off when I need a little breathing room and can swiftly revert back to multiple daily injections in the interim. (Especially since my doctor feels strongly about having all kinds of back-ups in place for pump failure, leaving me with the right tools for MDI.) Is pumping easier? For me, it is because I love micro-dosing (Correcting a blood sugar of 140 mg/dL back down to 100 without having to pierce my skin? Party time). And I appreciate the convenience of fluctuating basal rates and precision dosing.

Like I said—OPTIONS. I like knowing that, if I want to take a little bit of a break, for whatever reason, I'm armed with the tools and the data to go back and forth as I see fit. Diabetes doesn't afford me a lot of options (as in—"I'd love the option to send you the hell back to wherever you came from."), but I do have a choice in how I deliver my synthetic insulin, or what finger I prick for a blood sugar result, or which meter fits best into my life. Sometimes I need to take advantage of the opportunity to juggle, especially when I was so nervous about going the wearable technology route in the first place.

"*I think feeling nervous is a totally, totally normal reaction,*" said Kim. "*Everyone has to do what works for them. Give it a try, at least, but know that if an insulin pump or CGM doesn't work for you and your lifestyle, that's okay. Health isn't all glucose levels and insulin doses—it's about your mental health, too. You need to choose the tools that can help you achieve a healthy A1C, but also will help you be the happy and confident person with diabetes you're meant to be.*"

Karen found embracing the "it's not permanent" mentality to be what gave her the confidence to try a diabetes device or two. "*My endo said exactly the right thing when she said, 'It's not forever. If you hate it, you don't have to keep doing it.' It gave me the courage to try it out, and once I did, I never looked back. I feel so confident about my self-care right now. I have the data to help me fix things, I have a CGM that shows me trends that were hidden for years, I have a pump that lets me correct for a blood sugar of 130 mg/dL—it seems like a lot and it is, at first, but then a switch flips and all that gear makes diabetes seem a little easier.*"

Harry sums it up beautifully: "*I wish I could say that*

you're going to love it and you won't even notice it, but to be honest, I am completely aware that I have things attached to me and that my pockets will never be empty. It's easy to get hung up on that, and that's exactly why I resisted the idea of the pump for many years. What's hardest to see up front, though, is the benefit that those devices provide. It's difficult to put a value on getting a good night's sleep without waking up at a blood sugar of 300 mg/dL, or being able to spontaneously go for a long run if I unexpectedly have a free afternoon, but I know the pump and CGM give me the freedom to do these things."

Chapter Eleven

Bringing Your Diabetes to Work

I comb through job openings all the time because you never know when the urge to go down a new path will strike you. Being ready to apply includes a résumé polish, lint-rolling all the cat hair off my business suit (a daunting task), and preparing for the interview process.

And as a person with diabetes, preparing for an interview also includes the internal debate as to if, and when, it is best to let your employer know you have diabetes.

Safety is a top priority for me, and I'm not comfortable being involved in work or social situations without at least someone knowing I have diabetes. I want my employer to know that I have diabetes because that keeps me safest. If someone strolls by and sees me pale and almost passed out at my desk, I can't have them think I'm recovering from a wild night of unicycling. I need for diabetes to be the first thing they think of. I would much rather issue the "I'm Kerri and I have type 1 diabetes ..." educational speech than to need help and have no one aware of my health needs. The more people who know, the safer I am.

But what about an interview environment? Or even after a job is secured—when is the best time to tell? And are my rights protected in the workplace, as a person with diabetes?

Katie Hathaway, Managing Director, Legal Advocacy at the American Diabetes Association, views disclosure as a personal decision that varies from individual to individual. "*Whether to disclose your diabetes to an employer or potential employer is an entirely personal decision, and not one I can make for someone else. There are pros and cons to both choices. If you disclose your diabetes, you may find coworkers who are willing to help you if your blood glucose drops low and you need someone to get you a juice, or even to administer glucagon. Disclosing your diabetes is also necessary if you need an accommodation to do your job—for example, you sometimes experience hypoglycemia in the morning and need to arrive late to work. If your employer does not know that your late arrival is because of a disability, or you have not worked that out with your supervisor in advance, you could be at risk for discipline or even discharge. On the other hand, some people who either don't need accommodations or who do not want to risk discrimination if they disclose may choose to keep this information private. There is no wrong choice here.*"

Personally, I don't want anyone knowing I have diabetes until the deal is closed. When the interviewer looks at me, I want them to see a potential employee who is ready to give her all at the workplace, not a person whom they perceive as someone who will take extra sick days and will not be able to perform. People with diabetes are protected by the Americans with Disabilities Act and employers are not to discriminate against someone for having diabetes. I appreciate that legislation. However, I use extra caution.

Flashback to 2004: I check my blood sugar in the car before I go into a job interview. My meter reads 104 mg/dL. Below 150 mg/dL, for me, is too low for an interview, as I know that the more nervous I become, the faster my blood sugar may drop. I pop two glucose tabs into my mouth to take a preemptive strike against ill-timed hypoglycemia. I also switch the pump from "audible beep" to "vibrate" alarm mode and tuck it deep into my suit jacket pocket. No one knows I'm wearing a medical device. My medical alert bracelet is jangling on one arm, but it is discreet. My purse has my testing kit and a tube of glucose tabs for a just-in-case low. Upon meeting me, I look like a woman in pursuit of a job, without a whisper of evidence of diabetes.

The interview proceeds on its merry path, same as any other. They don't ask, because they can't, and I don't tell because diabetes doesn't affect my performance at work. Smiles were exchanged, an offer was made, and I'm hired.

It's not until my first or second day at work that I pull my new boss aside and tell them I have diabetes. "Just so you know, so I can feel safe," I offer.

They always respond with, "I'm glad you told me."

Sara Nicastro, who not only has type 1 diabetes but also a Masters of Education in College Student Affairs and has worked as a career counselor and academic advisor at a college, brings a perspective from both sides of the table. *"Disclosing diabetes or any disability is definitely a frequently asked question in the job search and career planning process. Employers are not allowed to discriminate against a candidate who has diabetes just like they are not allowed to discriminate based on gender, ethnicity, age, marital status, or any other protected class. As long as diabetes does not affect the candidate's ability to do the essential functions of the job, the employer does not have any right to know and a person with diabetes can choose to keep their diabetes private throughout the interview process and after being hired. On the other hand, if you can't be honest about yourself in an employment situation, and have to hide part of who you are, is that the right employment situation for you?"*

When it comes to disclosure, your diabetes preferences may vary (just as everything with diabetes seems to vary). Katie views disclosure in the workplace as a very personal decision, and one that is highly influenced by both the job itself and the openness of coworkers to understand diabetes. *"Some people who work in safety-sensitive jobs may be reluctant to go too far into the weeds of diabetes management for fear that a coworker will think they are unsafe to the job, and although decisions about whether a person's diabetes poses too big of a risk are not made by coworkers, it may be an annoyance one would rather not deal with. There is also the potential problem of over-policing by well-meaning coworkers. It's very much a balance between what you need them to know and what you feel comfortable with them knowing about you."*

Or perhaps what you feel comfortable with them assuming about you. Sara told me about an experience she had, where diabetes was mistaken as the root of an impassioned argument.

"At a different job, I was explaining to coworkers some of the common symptoms of both severe high and low blood sugars, and that when my blood sugar is low I often become irritable," Sara said. *"A few months later, I was discussing a situation with my director. We disagreed on the best approach to resolve the issues and I was passionately arguing my case. Apparently I was a little too passionate, because she said to me something like 'I think you need to go check your blood sugar. You are getting pretty upset about this.' I knew that my blood sugar was in range so it made me even angrier that she was blaming my passion on diabetes. I stormed back to my office and got out my meter. I still remember the result—93 mg/dL. I stomped back to her office with the meter in my hand. As I held the meter up to her face, I said, 'See. I'm not low. I'm just angry!'*

"While employers are not allowed to discriminate based on diabetes, you still want to be careful about the timing when you disclose it," said Sara, calling back her experience as a career counselor. *"The interview process should be a conversation. The candidate is finding out more information about the company at the same time that the company is finding out more information about the candidate. As long as your diabetes does not affect your physical ability to do your job, my advice on disclosure is to wait until after the offer of employment has been extended. That is the time in which you are finding out more about the insurance plans and other benefits of the company, so it makes sense to find out how your diabetes will fit with the organization. Depending on the size of the company, you are most likely dealing with human resources at this point as they process your paperwork, and not actually the people responsible for any hiring decisions. Think of it the same way as salary negotiation. You don't try to negotiate your salary in your first interview when they don't know anything about who you are and what you can do. It's better to wait until the company is convinced of your worth and will do anything to have you before you try to negotiate the benefits of your position. Once you have convinced them of your ability to do the job, your diabetes won't seem like anything more than a minor discussion point."*

I've never had trouble with the "when" of telling, but that balance between "telling" and "over-telling" is one I've struggled with throughout the years. I never want to make my diabetes seem like a reason why I wouldn't perform well at work, but at the same time, I wanted my employers and coworkers to understand that diabetes might require a little extra understanding at times. And sometimes, I may actually need someone's help.

A few years ago, I worked in the insurance industry in Rhode Island, as part of a large company in an office that housed approximately one hundred employees. My cubicle was near the front of the building, and the lunchroom was located at the far end of the building. I don't recall the specifics of what happened, but afterward, my coworker told me that I had gotten up from my desk, abruptly, and started walking toward the lunchroom. *"Only you weren't really walking, but more like staggering, touching your hand against the walls as you moved between the cubicles, like you were trying to hold yourself up. We got up to follow you, and when we caught up to you, it was clear that your blood sugar was in trouble."* Two of my coworkers helped get me to the lunchroom and bought a can of cranberry juice from the vending machine, urging me to drink it and sitting with me until I had consumed the contents of the can.

"For a few minutes, you weren't even looking at us. You were looking through us. But then, it was like the juice hit your system, and all of a sudden, you were back. And then you were fine. It was crazy, watching you tune back in like that. I can't even imagine where your brain was for those few minutes."

Even though I was embarrassed by the low, I was grateful for the quick and learned response of my coworkers. Because I had taken the time to explain low blood sugars and how to treat them, they were able to help me when I needed it. And that kind of safety net is worth a few minutes in a team meeting, explaining diabetes to them.

"I start out with the simple stuff when I explain diabetes to coworkers. I want them to know how to help in an emergency situation without being distracted by all the other details of living with diabetes," said Sara. *"I explain that emergency situations will usually occur when my blood sugar is too high or too low, but that an emergency when my blood sugar is too low is significantly more likely. I show them where my fast-acting sugar is and tell them to give that to me if I need help. The way I figure it, if my blood sugar is dangerously low, a little bit of sugar can save my life. If my blood sugar is dangerously high, that little bit of sugar is not going to make much of a difference. I would rather err on the side of a low blood sugar to be able to get the help that I need."*

To that same end, I made a "diabetes emergency kit" for when I worked in an office. In it were some diabetes-related supplies, such as backup infusion sets for my insulin pump and an insulin pen with fast-acting insulin, in case my pump was to fail at work. It also included a jar of glucose tabs and an emergency glucagon kit. I always instructed at least two people in my office to administer glucagon, if needed. (And

I always picked people I worked closely alongside. Actually, in one case, I picked the guy whose wife had type 1 diabetes, because he already knew all the necessary details.) And on the lid of the box, I wrote my "in case of emergency" phone numbers, including those of my mother and my husband, in the event that a family member needed to be alerted to a situation. It was kind of creepy, making that kit and taking into account all of the what-ifs that can happen throughout the day, but once it was completed and safely stashed at work, I felt prepared for the worst while I continued to assume the best.

And sometimes you don't even need to explain diabetes, because there are people who already understand. Sara told me about an experience she had where she wasn't the only diabetes community member in the room. "*I was interviewing for a job in Florida in September shortly after finishing graduate school. I had purchased a cute new skirt suit and was feeling pretty confident. My pump clipped securely to the waistband that made it quickly accessible at meal times but out of site from the potential interviewers. The interview had gone on all day. It was still pretty hot and humid in Florida at that point but I had managed to stay mostly inside and in the air conditioning. The last interview event of the day was dinner at a student festival on the large lawn in the center of campus, out in the blistering heat. I gathered my plate of food and sat at a table with the interview group.*

"*They were all pushing up their sleeves and fanning*

themselves to try to get relief from the heat as I sat there at the table in my suit jacket. My potential new boss repeatedly encouraged me to take my jacket off, but I tried to pretend that I wasn't hot. Then I tried to say I didn't want to take my jacket off because I only had a shell on underneath and it wasn't professional. She said that she didn't care, and that she just didn't want me to overheat. I knew that when I took my jacket off that my pump would be on full display and that I just would not be able to hide it. I couldn't handle the heat any longer and finally decided to give up the jacket. Of course my potential boss's eyes immediately went to the gray plastic clip on my waistband and I expected the worst. I was certainly surprised when she smiled and said, "Is that an insulin pump? My son has one, too."

Once the moments of disclosure are over, there are still concerns about diabetes management while on the job that need to be taken into consideration. How can a person with diabetes make sure that they have access to things such as glucose meters, snacks, etc. while still keeping in line with work policies?

"If you're referring to things such as access to food and drink, a place to test, etc., then I'd say it's up to each individual to make sure they have the accommodations they need to manage diabetes on the job—and to speak up for them when you don't have what you need," advised Katie. *"Each person needs to evaluate his/her own needs, the workplace culture and rules. Do you need to ask permission*

to leave your desk, or can you come and go freely? Do you need special permission to keep food nearby? Be familiar with ALL of your employer's policies—the ones that cover specific rules, the ones that may tell you how any accommodations should be requested, the ones that mention the company's antidiscrimination policies, and the ones that cover how to file a grievance, if needed. Then seek out what you need, document your requests, and contact the American Diabetes Association if you need help."

That is the key: We, as people with diabetes, are protected by the Americans with Disabilities Act of 1990. You have the right to manage your diabetes while doing your job, and the American Diabetes Association is on call—literally—to help people with diabetes assert and protect their rights.

If you feel that your rights in the workplace are being compromised, do not be afraid to reach out for help. *"The first step should be to call the American Diabetes Association at 1-800-DIABETES so we can provide you with some written materials and connect you with a legal advocate who can talk to you about your situation, discuss your legal rights, and connect you with other resources, such as lawyers in your area who can help you pursue your rights,"* said Katie. *"But there are other tips, too, such as making sure you write down everything that happens to you—even if you can't call us right away. It's incredibly helpful to keep a record of what is said, by whom, and what is done. And even though you don't need to call us right away—maybe you want to see how things develop—it's important to know that there are deadlines for taking legal action, and some deadlines can be short. The sooner you call, the sooner you can be helped.*"

Katie also recommends talking with your healthcare provider about providing a letter for your employer, documenting your need for certain accommodations. "*We have sample letters [on the ADA website] to help your healthcare provider with this. Other good resources are fellow people with diabetes, for moral support and practical experience with workplaces issues, referrals, and recommendations. And also your friends and family, because it can be hard to fight discrimination alone!*"

It can be a delicate balance of disclosure and maintaining your privacy, but in the end, your safety at work should be paramount. Do what makes you feel most comfortable, and don't be afraid to speak up on your own behalf.

Chapter Twelve

Diabetes and Exercise

Finding the motivation to exercise can be as challenging as the motivation to stay tuned in to diabetes. I think it's because there isn't an instant payoff. I walk out of the gym after one cardio session and I don't feel magically transformed. This frustration is similar to how a week of intense diabetes monitoring doesn't immediately drop my A1C. It's a slow burn toward seeing or feeling progress, and the lack of immediate results of all that hard work makes sticking with the program difficult, at times. (Versus the consumption of delicious cheeseburgers equaling instant and delicious gratification. Cruelly unfair.)

But the reminders as to why exercise is important are everywhere. Aside from the positive effect exercise has on my diabetes—improved cardiovascular health, increased muscle mass leading to a more efficient use of insulin, oh, and the handy fact that a 150 mg/dL can be brought down with a brisk walk faster than it can be fixed with a correction dose of insulin—exercise is important for overall health. Exercise isn't just for bringing down a high blood sugar and it's not just for people who have diabetes. Exercising your body is something that everyone, regardless of health status, should be attempting to do on a very regular basis. Sitting at the computer and writing e-mails? Necessary for work and financial survival. But going for a walk—or even a run—and getting your heart rate up and your blood flowing? That's necessary for the continuation of your life.

As a person with diabetes, I put an unfair amount of judgmental focus on my A1C level, or on the snapshot of a blood sugar result from my meter. These things matter—quite a bit—but there are a lot of other aspects of my health to take into consideration before stamping me with the seal of good health approval. What matters, in addition to these diabetes-related health obligations, is the total sum of my health. I still need to pay attention to the physical needs that matter to most bodies, not just our pancreatically challenged ones. Namely, exercise.

Chloe Vance, diagnosed with type 1 diabetes at the age of 18 and founder and executive director of the Connected in Motion organization, which focuses on diabetes and exercise in Canada, finds exercise to be a pivotal tool in her management arsenal. "*I know, without a doubt, that regular, moderate physical activity makes my diabetes way easier to manage. When I am on an outdoor adventure, however, I don't necessarily have the most stellar blood glucose results of all time. I keep my numbers in a range that enables me to get to my goals, live my life, and pursue my dreams safely. For me, living without the feeling that diabetes is holding me back from accomplishing my goals or dreams gives me the ability to have a much more positive outlook on diabetes and life in general."*

I spoke with Blair Ryan again for this one, as she is a lifelong athlete and deeply involved in the Insulindependence organization in San Diego, focused on diabetes and exercise. *"I am lucky that I was an athlete before I had diabetes, because for a long time running was my motivation for good control. In order to train and race well, I had to have good blood sugars. More recently, my life priorities have shifted and I spend most of my time and energy on my work, which involves a lot of time in front of a computer. I've found that maintaining good control is harder when I am not preparing for exercise at some point. On days without planned exercise, I don't eat as well, drink enough fluids, and sometimes am distracted from that pursuit of diabetes control. I am most motivated to manage my diabetes in the context of exercise. Exercise holds me accountable."*

I have to be honest—when I hear this kind of advice, I find myself nodding in agreement, but then I immediately wonder "Can I do this?" The desire to exercise, for me, is just as cyclical as diabetes burnout. There are months when I'm all,

"YES, EXERCISE, LET'S ALL DO THAT NOW!" and then there are months when I can't even find the caps button on the keyboard at all, let alone force myself to go outside to play.

During past moments of deep diabetes burnout, I didn't go to the gym without dragging myself there. (Literally. Like tying myself to the bumper of the car and putting a brick on the gas pedal, dragging myself down the road until I had hauled myself into the parking lot.) I went, but not with excitement or vigor or any kind of desire to do anything other than plod around on the treadmill and hit the predetermined mark so I could put the gold star on my mental chart.

So how can you get started, when the task may seem daunting, or if you are feeling unmotivated?

Chloe suggests taking the word *exercise* right out of your thought process. "*Don't think of it as exercise! Think about it simply as adding more activity to your daily routine. Can you walk or bike instead of drive? How about an hour outside instead of on Facebook? Start small and build up—the more successful positive exercise and activity experiences we have, the less scary it is.*"

Powerlifter and PWD Ginger Vieira agrees with the slow-and-steady approach. "*Pick one or two, maybe three, days of the week that you will go for a walk or go to a Zumba class. Staying fit affects everything—more than just my diabetes. It impacts how I feel as I walk down the street simply because when I'm exercising regularly, I feel in touch and connected with my own body. I feel aware of what my body can do, what it's capable of, and that makes me feel more confident in myself!*"

Slow and steady—I can do that. I have done that. For me, finding balance with diabetes and exercise meant first building the confidence to try new things. Exercise isn't something I'm shy about, but doing it in front of other people scares the hell out of me. I don't know why. I think it's because I've been blessed with such a high level of extreme awkwardness that the thought of doing anything in front of people makes me freeze up. I didn't want to walk down the aisle at my own wedding for fear of tripping and falling. (I wanted to furtively rise up on a platform from underneath the floor, like an elevator, and just appear at the front of the church to say "I do!") I am nervous about going from my table to the podium when I speak at events. So the idea of crossing a finish line with an audience and an event photographer made me wish I was a Wonder Twin and could morph into "shape of innocuous shrubbery!" or something, last minute.

After years of working out in the confines and anonymity of a large gym, I wanted to break out of that rut and be outside, doing something new. I've been involved in some kind of exercise-related activity for most of my life. As a kid, I played soccer (badly), performed in tap-dance recitals (less badly, but more spandex and glitter, which was oddly worse), and rode my bike all over our neighborhood. During college, my roommates and I would go for walks down by the seawall along the ocean. And once I met my gym-centric husband, going to the gym became part of a normal day.

But these activities were all taking place privately, so to speak. No finish line. No cameras. No real audience (unless you count the dance recitals, which I'm desperately trying to forget).

Which is why it was a big deal, to me, to participate in my first official 5K race (meaning where there were other people and a start/finish line and people were wearing bibs with numbers instead of lobsters on them).

"I'm really proud of you for doing something that is so far outside your comfort zone," my husband said, and that's exactly it. That's why I felt compelled to follow through. A few of my runner friends have these T-shirts they wear, boasting about a race they completed, and I wanted to earn a T-shirt, too. I started attempting to run a few months back, and, at the beginning, finishing a mile without stopping or pitching backwards off the treadmill was a big accomplishment for me. Since that first attempt, I had built up some endurance and wanted to try the 3.1 mile race with the aim to finish, without walking and without falling into a ditch.

So far outside of my comfort zone that I couldn't even see the hazy edge, I proudly crossed the finish line. I didn't walk. I didn't come in last. My pace was decent. My blood sugars didn't tank. I felt proud of myself for following through on this, and not backing out in the end because I was self-conscious. And now I have a T-shirt that I earned.

But it wasn't just a matter of physically moving my body from point A to point B. I needed to also make sure my blood sugars weren't on an excursion of their own. My attempt at a 5K was accomplished, successfully, by training a lot. Not just training myself to run well, but also training my diabetes to keep up. It was a learning process for my body and my mind, and sometimes it was really hard. And on occasion, it was a bit scary.

"*Fear often comes from the unknown and the unpredictability of diabetes, especially during exercise,*" offered Chloe. "*I will admit that I've been caught alone, in the woods, dropping into a bad low blood sugar with all the food in a pack at the opposite end of the trail. That was scary. I learned from that experience. I'm not scared when I am prepared and have what I need to manage diabetes at my fingertips.*

"*So be prepared,*" Chloe said. "*Make sure you have your diabetes supplies with you. Check often, to know where your blood sugars are at, where they've been, and where they are going. Carry snacks and fast-acting glucose. But also exercise, and get outside with friends who know your needs so that they can watch your back.*"

Ginger truly does treat diabetes and exercise like a science experiment, fusing her knowledge about powerlifting with her personal experience living with diabetes. "*When I first started becoming more active and pursuing powerlifting, I decided I wasn't going to let diabetes fluctuations get in the* way of my athletic goals. I viewed every workout as an experiment. I wrote down what I ate, how much insulin I took, what kind of workout I did, and the impact on my blood sugar. My inspiration came from my goal to be successful.

"Now, when I start a new type of exercise, I eat the same thing before each time I do that exercise. I write down my pre-exercise blood sugar. I consume 15 grams of carbs without insulin to start on the safe side for preventing lows. I check my blood sugar halfway through to see how things are going, and at the end, as well. If I'm low by the end of my routine, then I know I need more carbs, or less insulin. If I'm high, then I know the workout was more anaerobic and, therefore, didn't use glucose for fuel but utilized more body fat instead. I then re-create that whole experiment several times over to build my confidence in the plan.

"Today, through experiments and learning the basics of exercise physiology, I understand that I can easily prevent lows and burn more body fat for fuel by doing more anaerobic style workouts—any type of strength training, high-intensity burst training, and sprints or interval style cardio— and I actually need to take a smidge of insulin to prevent the highs that naturally come with these types of exercise," added Ginger. "Exercising first thing in the morning on an empty stomach, without any carbs but sometimes with an extra smidge of insulin, and an in-range starting blood sugar is also a really easy way to work out while burning body fat for fuel rather than glucose."

And Blair views exercise as a way to make diabetes more forgiving and less of an all-consuming focus. *"I strive to devote as little brainpower to diabetes as possible, while maintaining good control. Exercise minimizes the time I spend thinking about diabetes. For me, the clearest examples of this were when I ran competitively in high school and college, and I'd have 14 days off a year. It never failed that during those two weeks I'd need to increase my basal rate, bolus more, and count carbohydrates more precisely. The relative ease that exercise brings to my diabetes management is enough to get me out of bed or out the door after work. I crave endorphins, and I am thankful that exercise is crucial to diabetes management. If exercise truly complicated diabetes management, I'd be in a terrible place."*

I will admit to not embracing my inner mad scientist when working through my exercise process, but I do try to mitigate as many variables as possible. For me, exercise creates a heightened anxiety about low blood sugars. Before I head out for a run, I try hard to make sure I don't have any active insulin in my system (no recent bolus, no insulin on board [IOB] on my pump). I keep a tube of glucose tabs tucked into my running belt, and I always have my continuous glucose monitor close to my body, so that I can feel any vibrations alerting me to highs or lows. And the ubiquitous cell phone, which I say is for listening to running playlists, but is more for an emergency situation in the event that I need to call for help. Being prepared makes me feel like the worst that can happen is planned for, and the best that can happen is that I'll beat my time.

When I'm exercising at the gym, I'm usually by myself (absent people who know me and my diabetes, that is—the gym itself is usually packed with strangers), so I make a point to tell the people who work at the gym that I have diabetes. This isn't an awkward discussion I have every time I visit, but a chat I've had once, when signing up for the gym. I ask the folks who work there to mark my profile as "type 1 diabetic," so that if something were to happen, it would be on their radar. Knowing they have that knowledge, in addition to the medical alert bracelet I wear while working out, makes me feel safe. That feeling of safety helps me actually enjoy the workout.

Because there are times when I need someone to know. There was one instance when I had walked out of the gym after exercising and checked my blood sugar before driving home. The result on the meter shocked me, as I didn't have a single low symptom, other than a slight headache. But seeing that 35 mg/dL staring back at me was enough to move me from the car and back into the safety of the gym, where there were people who could help, if the situation became more than I could handle.

The guy at the counter was checking in some new members, but he looked twice at me as I grabbed a bottle of orange juice from the cooler and leaned heavily on the counter, downing the majority of the bottle in a few gulps.

"You okay?" he asked.

"Sort of. I'm having a very low blood sugar moment right now and I didn't want to sit in my car alone, in case there was a problem." I tried to smile, but I was so jerky and unsteady that I resembled a hungry dinosaur more than a woman. All teeth, stretched smile, and my eyes were trying to find something that was roughly 1,000 yards away.

"Okay. We'll wait until you're up again." He finished signing in the new members and I tried to convince myself I was at a bar instead of the gym. ("*How you doin'? Sure, you can buy me a ... a bottle of juice.*")

For about 15 minutes, the gym guy chatted with me about how diabetes—both type 1 and type 2—has infiltrated his family. Grandmothers on both sides, aunts, cousins, his sister, his father, and his mom ... the list of affected family went on for the duration of my low blood sugar. So many members of his family were dealing with some version of this disease. He knew exactly how diabetes could ruin your day. And he could see how it was making a mess of those few moments for me.

"I am sorry for taking up so much of your time. I feel much better now. Thanks for keeping an eye on me." I said, embarrassed, but back up to 98 mg/dL and feeling more human.

"Any time. You were exercising your right to loiter," he said. "It's a good way to cool down after a workout, right?"

Working out with the confidence I'm in safe, knowledgeable company makes exercising less of a nerve-wracking chore and more of something to which I even (sort of?) look forward. Because after that workout is over? I feel better. Even if it was a tough workout, and even if my blood sugars weren't exactly playing nice, I am drafting off the endorphins and proud that I put my body through the paces.

Ginger seconded that sentiment, saying, *"The more active I am, the more motivated I am to eat healthy foods and check my blood sugars more often, because being active has this sneaky way of making you want to do healthier things for yourself in other areas of your life. Staying fit, staying in shape, and moving my body makes me feel like diabetes can't stop me from accomplishing anything. 'Look, diabetes, I can jump rope like Rocky Balboa! You ain't got nothin' on me!'"*

Exercising with diabetes isn't so much about balance as it is about perseverance. "Don't stop, don't give up," becomes a mantra that runs through my mind when I'm pushing myself through a hard workout. Diabetes makes moving your body tougher with all of its variables—blood sugar fluctuations, insulin levels, carb impact, etc.—but having diabetes is even more of a reason to move. I used to be great at making up excuses: too busy, too tired, too low, too high, too bored, too uninspired. My brain was trained to blurt out excuses for avoiding exercise. My exercise routine was a sad state of affairs, and my body paid the price with a higher body mass index (BMI) and fluctuating A1Cs. After realizing that my stress levels, blood sugars, and pants sizes could all be lowered with the help of some good old-fashioned running around, I set my mind to achieve a fitter state of mind and body.

There are still moments of frustration, where my body and my numbers aren't in tune, but I keep moving forward. This is the only body I'll have, and it deserves my respect, determination, and constant push toward good health.

Chapter Thirteen

Finding Balance in Trains, Planes, and Automobiles

In the last few years, I've done a considerable amount of traveling. This was after a long drought of not going anywhere, for fear of the unknown and pretty much everything else, but now I'm constantly on the move. Whether for work or for fun, or a combination of both, this means a lot of air travel and plenty of not-being-home.

I wish I were a more fluid traveler (maybe I should try more boats?), but I'm not. I'm painfully high strung when it comes to preparing for a few days on the road. Years ago, I would bring a suitcase big enough to stow away a small horse, but since traveling more frequently, I've learned to streamline the process (and to leave the horse behind). Of course, I always play the "What did I forget" game when I'm about to walk out the door, or while I'm on that anxiety-inducing ride to the airport, where I convince myself that

I left my cell phone/pump/license/head/house keys at home and I have to keep checking, repeatedly, to ensure the safety of these items. (Not even once have I forgotten my head, despite my mother's constant threats of it being left behind, were it not attached.)

What makes preparing such a process are the health-centric decisions. Whether I'm in Philadelphia for two days or in London for a week, I bring backups of my backups. Three-day trip? Three new infusion sets. Three bottles of test strips. A brand-new bottle of insulin. The in-case-of-pump-failure insulin pen. And let's not forget the normal essentials, like socks. All this baggage does not a light suitcase make.

And after speaking with several other people with diabetes who are on the move more often than not, I realized I wasn't alone in my traveling tendencies. Many of my fellow travelers with diabetes plan ahead and pack carefully.

"*In my teens and twenties, I traveled back and forth to Europe for vacations. In my thirties, I became a 'road warrior' for my job, often flying coast to coast ... or to places less glamorous. I've also done my share of road-tripping, heading to destinations 10 to 18 hours away,*" said Christel Aprigliano, type 1 since the age of 12.

Dana Lewis, a twenty-something living in the Pacific Northwest, has also logged her share of miles, in addition to years with type 1 diabetes. "*When I was the American Diabetes Association National Youth Advocate in 2006–2007, I traveled to a dozen diabetes camps in a single summer, and other events around the country during the rest of the year. I've flown to international conferences in South Africa, Germany, Hungary, and Spain. I traveled to New Jersey for an internship one summer and lived out of two suitcases for two months. I've traveled to many an uninteresting conference room around the United States for various health-care conferences, as well."*

Dana has also braved the backpacking route, living out of a backpack for a month. *"I spent 31 days in Europe in the summer of 2010, visiting 11 countries and living out of a single backpack. I also cross the country several times a year to visit my family in the southeast, since I'm currently residing in Seattle."*

The idea of backpacking across a continent impresses and intimidates me as a newly comfortable traveler. Packing obsessively is a part of my travel routine from which I can't deviate. Regardless of where I'm going, all this health stuff comes along with me. It makes for a long mental packing list. It makes me test the limits of airline carry-on policies. (It probably puts me on a no-fly list in some circumstances.)

How do you make sure you have what you need, in terms of both diabetes and non-diabetes supplies? *"Test often—and pack survivor-style,"* said Dana. *"For me, the key is being prepared with enough pump supplies, test strips, and food to be able to weather just about anything for the duration of my trip. This also means I pack plenty of snacks in case*

I can't find food to eat for meals—I'm gluten-free because of celiac disease—and more juice boxes than a sane person would haul around in her carry-on. Being prepared has helped me combat lows while hiking in Switzerland; riding a bike around Amsterdam; geo-caching in South Africa; and dragon boating in the Pacific Northwest."

Christel borrows from the "be prepared!" mentality, especially when it comes to circumstances outside of our control. "*Always keep something to eat in your carry-on, briefcase, purse, and/or person. You might think you'll grab something in the terminal before you board your flight, but sometimes— often—things don't go as planned. Even a granola bar can help stave off hunger and a potential low blood sugar. I've been stuck on the tarmac for a few hours waiting for the weather to clear, and believe me, those peanuts don't feel filling. And do I need to mention the importance of carrying glucose tabs? Should go without saying.*"

The night before I leave for any trip, I make sure I'm fully packed. That way, any last-minute panicky moments can happen in time to find the solution. This includes packing up my medical supplies and making sure they fit into my carry-on bag. My carry-on includes my glucose meter, glucose tablets, a backup pump infusion set, replacement batteries for my meter and pump, a spare continuous glucose sensor, test strips, and any vials of insulin. I keep my spare glucose meter in my checked luggage, but everything else stays with me and within reach.

Christel also keeps the majority of her supplies in her carry-on, for easier access. "*I don't put diabetes supplies in my luggage if I'm packing for a trip less than a week. It all goes in a duffel bag carry-on. I just don't trust baggage handlers to get my bags from one place to the next, and I speak from experience. All my medications go into a clear bag like you would with liquids. All my pump supplies, CGM supplies, and test strips go into the duffel along with a slew of glucose tabs and a box of granola bars or snack food that I'm sure I'll want to eat in my hotel room at some point.*"

"*I always carry a minimum of a bottle of insulin, syringes, test strips, and a pump site and reservoir in my carry-on,*" agreed Dana. "*I also do a little overkill in the juice department and carry 8 to 10 juice boxes with me, even if I'm only on a two-hour flight, and snacks to last for a meal or two. I also always try to carry an extra pump clip, because armrests on airplanes eat pump clips for breakfast.*"

Insulin pump issues are a concern of mine while traveling, as well. While I assume my pump will work just fine, I prefer to have an insulin pen or two in my bag, in case my pump has any issues while I'm on the move. Usually I request a "loaner pump" from my insulin pump company as a backup while I travel. I also confirm that I have enough fast-acting insulin, back-up basal insulin, syringes, and test strips for the trip well ahead of time, in case I need to get new prescriptions from my medical team.

There's also the mental dance of when to change the time setting on my pump. My basal rates remain steady throughout the day, except for a few hours in the morning when they're cranked up to almost triple the normal amount to take a bite out of the dawn phenomenon that I've experienced for years. That pesky "wake up at 80 mg/dL but then go up to 200 mg/dL for no effing reason" phenomenon. That "midnight to 5 AM at 0.45 units, then all the way up to 0.85 units at 5 AM until 9:30 AM, when it goes back down to 0.45 units" mess.

It's definitely part of the reason an insulin pump works for me, because without the ability to tweak that morning basal rate, I'd be dealing with highs that frustrate me endlessly since they aren't the product of breakfast or stress. They just *are*. I like being able to keep things steady, especially when I'm away from home and at the mercy of schedules, time changes, and other travel concerns.

I forget, though, how important that basal crank is for me. I take basal bump from the pump for granted sometimes, because once it's programmed, it's not something I think about. It's not until I travel outside of my time zone that I have to start juggling the dosing details again, making me run low at strange times of the day until my body clock adjusts to whatever time zone I'm in.

Usually, I change the time on my pump as soon as the plane reaches cruising altitude, and I try to adjust to the local time zone as soon as possible. One time, for the first time ever, I forgot to change my pump on the ride home. And then neglected to change it back for several days, until I looked at my pump at 11 AM and saw it claiming 5 AM. Which explained the weird, ill-timed highs that week in the morning hours and the strange double-down arrows at lunchtime.

Being prepared is important, especially when you are traveling alone. For trips where my husband or a friend is traveling with me, I bring a glucagon injection kit, in case of severe hypoglycemia, but in most instances, I'm on my own and responsible for my own care. My medical alert bracelet is marked as a necessity for travel. As a person with type 1 diabetes, low blood sugars are always an unnerving threat, and they can sneak up on me without warning. If my blood sugar were to tumble into hypoglycemia range, what would happen if I were to pass out? People would see a woman who was passed out, and would have no idea that diabetes could be in play. Paramedics (and people, in general) are trained to be on the lookout for medical alert jewelry, more so than they are trained to be aware of insulin pumps and glucose meters. Although I've never lost consciousness due to a low blood sugar, I have had moments when I've been unable to effectively communicate, and the power of simply pointing to my wrist has, perhaps, saved my life.

As far as low glucose treatments, my weapon of choice remains the glucose tab, for several reasons. One is that they are perfectly portioned out to help me treat a low without over-treating. I can chomp down four of them and know that

I've safely consumed 16 grams of fast-acting carbs. And they keep me from over-treating because they don't taste as awesome as a fistful of jelly beans, helping me consume only what needs to be consumed. Lastly, they don't melt. Or freeze. (They seem impervious and could possibly survive an apocalyptic event.) They also aren't liquid, so there isn't any added Transportation Security Administration (TSA) concern when trying to get them through security points.

"*Wear your medical alert bracelet/necklace/tattoo in plain sight,*" cautions Christel. "*It may not be sexy, but traveling is stressful and if something happens to you and you can't communicate, it's the only thing that may help you. Keep emergency contact information in your wallet or on your phone and use the ICE acronym—In Case of Emergency— next to the person's name. Thankfully, I've never experienced any diabetes-related travel incidents, which, considering how much I'm on the road, is a triumph in itself.*"

Dana has dealt with a few issues while traveling, but mostly related to airport security. "*My biggest disasters have been with TSA, and luckily those weren't true disasters as much as a test of patience and my ability to argue to the letter of the law about federal guidelines of medical liquids in your carry-on. It seems like every time I travel—even through the same airports—TSA regulations have changed as to how they check medical liquids and/or the TSA agents are more or less educated about medical devices and medical liquids, so I'm always on my toes and speaking clearly and firmly about my rights as a traveler with diabetes in order to make sure I get all of my supplies—including a bag filled with juice boxes— onto the plane with me."*

Also, it can be helpful to have a letter from your doctor, explaining that you have diabetes and noting some of the items you may be required to have on you while you travel. For domestic travel, you might not ever pull the letter out, but if you are in a place where you don't speak the language, a letter in the local language can help you navigate questions about things like glucose meters and insulin pumps.

I've experienced my share of airport security checkpoints over the years, and most of the time, it hasn't been a big issue. Usually, the TSA agent has seen a pump before and just needs a little background on the Dexcom, which I'm happy to give. Airport security doesn't work me up. I'm not shy, and I'm not easily rattled about the screenings, so I'm fine with waiting patiently for the "female assist!!" to show up and examine my devices by hand and screening wand.

But I do remember, and assert, the fact that I have rights. I have the right to opt out of the TSA body scanners. I have the right to stand there, politely, and wait for someone to manually inspect my diabetes devices. I have the right to decline to send my medical devices through the scanning machines. I don't make unreasonable demands during airport security screenings, and I follow the rules as they are laid out to me. In return, I hope for and am not shy about demanding respect when the TSA agents are examining my personal belongings and my physical body. (I also keep a close watch on my CGM graph, because it's almost comical to watch it spike up after apologizing my way through the security checkpoints.)

Managing diabetes on the road sometimes means pulling a few tricks out of your sleeve or from the hotel minibar. When I'm on the road, the Dexcom continuous glucose monitor is the safety net I need to feel safe about sleeping at night. Trouble is, sometimes I don't hear the alarms coming from the receiver when I need to most. How good is a CGM you can't hear? (Answer: not terribly) To make the alarm louder and jarring enough to wake me up, I take a glass from the minibar and put my Dexcom receiver in it while I sleep. The sound of the CGM vibrating and beeping from the glass is loud and enough to rouse me from a deep sleep, or a troubling low.

"My latest diabetes hack has been a giant Ziploc bag full of supplies that I keep stashed in my favorite travel bag," said Dana. *"When I travel, whether it's a weekend or overnight trip, or hopping on a plane for a cross-country trip, I simply grab that bag as my first packed item to make sure that I have backup sites, reservoirs, test strips, syringes, allergy medication, etc. I pack plenty of supplies for each trip's duration, but if you are running out the door or making a quick grab for an overnight bag, there's comfort in knowing that you have one or two of everything you could possibly need in one bag in the same place, and that your basics are covered. This*

bag includes some of the less common things that I might use like Zofran [to help curb nausea] and other things that come in handy for travel.

"My less exciting hack is usually buying a regular soda at the airport when I land at my final destination, and taking it with me to the hotel so I don't have to worry about digging my juice out from the bottom of my bag for a late-night/early-morning travel low. I know I've got extra sugar at hand in case my juice supply is running low from the flight."

But it's not all about dealing with emergencies and worrying about the circus-esque experience that traveling with a medical condition can become. It's also about exploring new places, and having fun seeing what's outside your own zip code.

"My biggest triumph was that backpacking trip. Thirty-one days, with a single backpack," said Dana. (When I heard that, I was wholly impressed because my daily purse is the size of a backpack. Dana mastered some truly streamlined packing!) *"Granted, there were plenty of sodas for lows bought in foreign languages, but having enough glucose tabs and snack bars to combat a number of days without food—in case I didn't trust my language skills in interpreting 'gluten-free' in half a dozen languages—and lows from walking 10 plus miles a day or hiking through Switzerland was key. I'm also proud that I was, and still am, able to travel by myself and deal with any situation, whether it's a high or*

low blood sugar, or stepping off the train in a country where I don't speak the language. Having enough supplies and a plan for any diabetes-related disasters will help you no matter what situation you're in so you can rely on habit as to where your supplies are stashed, and know they're there when you need them."

For me, I reached a new level of confidence with traveling and diabetes when I found myself traveling alone to the Middle East for a diabetes conference. As a place I'd never anticipated having the opportunity to visit, it was an incredibly liberating experience going somewhere so far, and so different, from my day-to-day culture exposure. I navigated a completely new world without panicking (that lack of panic was new for me). Almost seven thousand miles from home, I felt oddly confident. To people who have been comfortable traveling their whole lives, this isn't a big deal. But for me, this was a big deal. Plenty of people travel that far away every day. And there are millions of people far more traveled than me. But that trip, in particular, really opened my eyes to the fact that the diabetes community has brought me to some incredible places and has given me the opportunity to cross things off of a list I didn't even realize I had.

Chapter Fourteen

Advocacy Outside of the Bubble

Diabetes advocacy isn't always about standing at a podium and giving a big, important speech to a room full of people. Sometimes the most powerful advocacy moments happen during dinner meetings, or in line at the grocery store.

"*I have family members with diabetes, but they don't take care of themselves,*" said one of the guys at our dinner meeting. "*They eat whatever they want, and they never test their blood sugar, and they never go to the doctor.*"

The unspoken thought, capping the end of that sentence, felt like, "So they deserve whatever they get."

The others at my dinner table were aware of the fact that I have type 1 diabetes, but it wasn't a big discussion point throughout the day, so I think it was a little snippet of information that fell by the wayside by the time dinner was served. But even though I was at this dinner with people

I didn't really know, and who didn't really know me, I couldn't control the urge to speak up.

"But how do you know that?" I blurted out.

He stopped and looked at me. "What do you mean?"

"How do you know they don't take care of themselves? Or go to the doctor? Or check their blood sugar?"

"Because they don't. I never see it. Not even at holidays."

I didn't want to be "That Person." I had zero desire to be the one who raises her voice at a dinner table with strangers, preaching on about the misconceptions society has about diabetes, and about all the different types of people who live with it, and on and on. I wanted to have dinner and hang out, having a good time.

But I don't like the "but the majority of people with diabetes DON'T take care of themselves" argument, because I take care of myself. I try and I do. And I know so many people who take care of themselves the best they can, and so many who, despite dedicated efforts, still run a rough road. Perfection isn't achievable, and guilt is inescapable. My husband encourages me to not take these discussions personally, because he hates to see my feelings hurt, but it's hard not to take it personally. I have diabetes. They're talking about diabetes. Even when I try, it's hard to keep my viewpoints objective.

"Did you see me check my blood sugar at the table a few minutes ago?"

"You did?"

"Yeah. I have checked twice, actually, at this table. While you sat there. And that orange juice I had before? Which might not have seemed like the 'right' food for a diabetic? I was treating a low blood sugar. You don't always see what we do to take care of ourselves. But there's a lot that we do. I swear." I smiled at him, but inside I was begging, pleading for him to see me as a person who, however my life wrings out, didn't "deserve" a damn thing.

There was an awkward silence.

"Twice? You tested twice?"

"Yeah."

This time, he smiled warmly, erasing all awkwardness. "Maybe they do stuff I don't see, too."

I smiled back, relieved, now trying to control the urge to hug him.

"I hope so."

Type 1 diabetes isn't something you can see readily. It's not an illness that, at this point in my life, comes with any constant external symptoms. I am fortunate enough to not use a wheelchair or need vision-assistance devices. You can't see my disease, even though it's something I manage every day. Type 1 diabetes is a chronic illness, and one that has required daily maintenance and effort from me, and from my caregivers, for the last 27 years. Every morning starts with my meter. Every meal I've eaten in the last two plus decades has been preceded by a blood sugar check and an insulin dose. And every night has my finger pricked by a lancet before my head hits the pillow.

This isn't a pity party. Not by a long shot. My life is healthy and I have a very fulfilling existence, even if days are bookended by diabetes and even if I'm now wearing medical devices 24 hours a day, every single day. Back when I was a fresh-faced kid, people seemed to want to cure my disease because they didn't like the idea of a small child dealing with such a big disease. Kids have futures that seem hard not to invest in.

But doesn't everyone have a future worth investing in? Type 1 diabetes became a part of my life a long time ago, and I don't remember even a snippet of "the before." Even though I've lived very well with this disease and kept myself from feeling owned by it in any way, it's still here. And it's still something I deal with every day, regardless of how well or poorly controlled. But just because I'm no longer a little kid with the bright, shining future, am I any less diabetic? Any less deserving of that cure? Just because you can't see my disease, and because I seem to have it under physical and emotional control, does not mean it's past the point of deserving a cure.

This is why I advocate. Whether it seems invisible or not, diabetes is very visible to me, to so many people I care about, both young and old. I want to help raise awareness for diabetes to help improve the lives of people living with it and caring for it.

I wasn't always involved in diabetes advocacy efforts, and

neither was my family. "*To be honest, we heard about the promise of a cure right at the outset*," said my mother, discussing our efforts toward diabetes advocacy back in 1986. "'*In five years, there will be a cure. They are so close,' is what we heard from doctors and national advocacy groups. That kind of mentality makes you think, 'If I just hold on tight for five more years, it will be gone.' Back then, we were headed down the 'five more years' path, and it was near impossible to think that they were wrong, or that they may have lied to us. I remember feeling discouraged. I wonder if I'd have been a better advocate had I known how long it would be.*"

My mother did search for support and community; it just wasn't very easy to find. "*Right after you were diagnosed, we went to a support group for parents of young kids with diabetes. It took place at Joslin, and it was the only support group I ever went to,*" my mother said. "*Back then, the Internet wasn't a readily available tool for finding others living with diabetes, or taking care of it, and not having access to any people made support nonexistent. But you didn't seem upset about not being part of a bigger support team. Diabetes was so much of your life as it was; we didn't want to focus even more on it. Besides, knowing you, you would have told us if you wanted to be involved. You were very vocal about what you wanted, and didn't want, in terms of your disease.*"

"*When I was diagnosed at the age of 17, just before I started my senior year of high school, the only thing I received that talked about community or advocacy of any kind was a paper telling me how I could sign up to be part of the ADA [American Diabetes Association],*" said George Simmons, who has been living with type 1 for more than 20 years. "*Other than that, nothing. No diabetes walks, no fundraisers, no coffee meet-ups for me or my mom. But honestly, that was okay with me at the time because the last thing I wanted to focus on was diabetes. I wanted to focus on being a drum major, graduation, and finding a girlfriend.*"

The defining moment for George, one that thrust him into the world of diabetes advocacy, was being admitted to the hospital. "*The catalyst was going to the hospital with diabetic ketoacidosis [DKA] back in 2005. That experience scared me straight and made me want to be educated about my diabetes. When I got home from that hospital stay, I started looking up podcasts about diabetes. I found one called DiabeticFeed, and it was hosted by a woman with type 1 diabetes who talked about diabetes. And on one show, she was interviewing a woman who wrote a blog about type 1 diabetes. I logged on, began to read, and realized I was not alone.*"

Christel Aprigliano, creator of DiabeticFeed and living with type 1 diabetes since she was 12 years old, was also looking to find others like herself. "*I had this realization that, in my mid-thirties, I didn't know anyone else who was going through the same things I was going through, as it related to diabetes. I didn't have anyone to talk to, to compare notes with. There was nothing out there from another person with diabetes's perspective. I talked with my boyfriend, and he told me to start a podcast. I had listened to some podcasts in the past, but none had anything to do with diabetes. My boyfriend had a background in radio and technology, so for him, it was a project we could work on together. I went the podcast route because no one else was doing it at the time."*

There's no one set way to advocate for diabetes. And being an advocate for diabetes doesn't need to fall within some kind of formal definition. With all these diabetes blogs, fundraising walks, speakers, and meet-up organizers, there's a lot going on in the world of diabetes awareness and community. Reach out to your local Juvenile Diabetes Research Foundation (JDRF) or American Diabetes Association (ADA) chapters, or even local hospitals and endocrinologist offices to see if they have in-person support groups set up, and if they don't, consider starting one yourself. Diabetes organizations and advocacy chapters are powerful resources in the quest to connect with others in the diabetes community. The Internet, as stated throughout this book, is a tremendous resource for finding others, taking away limitations such as zip codes and travel costs. If you're able to log on to the Internet, simply typing the phrase "diabetes blogs" or "diabetes community" into a search engine will provide instant connections.

Even with all of those opportunities, you don't have to blog or attend events or raise thousands for walk teams. You can raise a lot of awareness in what may feel like the smallest of ways, and you can make a real difference for just one person simply by connecting with them.

"*Realizing you aren't alone empowers you to learn more about diabetes and more about what life could be,*" said George, reflecting on the power of community. "*Online, in this community, there aren't any taboo topics. People were talking about everything, and learning, too. New medicines, new technologies, new specialists to see ... prior to going online and finding the diabetes community, I didn't even know I should have been seeing a specialist. These discussions really opened my eyes to the care I should be getting, but wasn't.*

"*We, as people with diabetes, need to reach more people. There needs to be a way to get to the people who feel like they are alone. Peeling back the loneliness shows an immediate health benefit—I'm proof! Through becoming involved with people who understand diabetes and what it's like to live with it, my A1C went from 12.5% to 10% in a month, and two months after that, it was already down to 8.3%. What changed? It was so simple—I learned that I should be checking my blood sugar two hours after I ate to see what my number was. So simple, but so true. Making that small change, and being dedicated to it, made a huge difference in my health.*"

Christel has stepped in and out of the diabetes space, both online and off, but the desire to connect with other people with diabetes has spanned the course of her lifetime with the disease. "*I wanted to share the real life stuff. Sometimes it's just the minutiae, and some of it's the tough stuff I wish other people would share. Like diabulimia—it needs to be talked about. I don't talk about it much, but when I do, I feel better. The things that people need to hear need to be talked about.*

"*Advocacy for me now takes a lot of different forms. I've helped to diagnose people,*" Christel said, remembering a time when a coworker approached her about health symptoms he'd been experiencing. "*He said, 'Hey, you know, I have some questions. I've been drinking a lot of water, and peeing, and I know it's summer and it's hot …' And I started to run down the symptoms to him, to see what he'd say yes to. The weight loss, the thirst, the peeing in the middle of the night. He said yes to so many.*

"'*Would you be willing to let me test you?' I pulled out a fresh lancet. His blood glucose was 374 mg/dL. He was diagnosed with type 2 diabetes soon thereafter, at an appointment with his doctor. Had he not felt like he could talk to me, he would have kept it to himself and things could have gotten really bad for him.*"

George touched upon the challenge of disclosure, even when you're eager to connect with others. "*It can be hard to find the confidence to share your health because it's so personal. Maybe people want to be involved, but they want to keep it low-key. Remember that every time you tell anyone about your diabetes life, you speak on behalf of a lot of people, and even a little education goes a long way. There's no pressure, but you should know you are doing a great service to the community when you share something about diabetes. When you correct a diabetes myth, you are doing the entire community a favor. That small act of education can make a huge ripple effect of awareness. You don't need to sign up or log in. You just need to share, in whatever way you're comfortable."*

But it can be hard, and even downright daunting, to think about sharing a personal health condition with strangers. Whether you're meeting with new people at a local coffee shop or entering a discussion in an online social network, it can be scary to make that first leap of sharing. For me, living in a quiet town in the smallest state, my ability to network with other people with diabetes is limited by my zip code, leaving the Internet as my go-to source for fellow PWDs. But for others who are living in a more PWD-populated area, in-person meet-ups and advocacy events are more likely. Regardless of how or when, I think it's so important for people living with and caring for people living with diabetes to find one another and connect. There's so much power to removing the isolation of diabetes.

Finding others can be a little intimidating and can feel like you're putting yourself out there to dangle in the wind. How do you find your community and become part of it? *"The key is to communicate, in any and every way you know how,"* said George. *"There are so many people sharing their stories now that finding someone in a similar life place as you could be easy. When you find that someone, initiate a con-versation. It can be scary—it does take a little stepping out on your part—but the payoff is amazing. With a little bit of searching, you can find that all-important kindred spirit. Go to a #dsma* [diabetes social media advocacy twitter chat] *chat and say, 'I am newly diagnosed and I don't know any type 1s,' and I guarantee you would get followers and people messaging you trying to connect."*

"*There also shouldn't be a pressure to become a certain kind of advocate,*" said my mom. "*There just shouldn't. No one should accuse you of not doing enough, saying things like, 'You don't want to champion for your child's disease?' Never forget that every parent, and every caregiver, supports their loved one. They advocate for the person with diabetes in their life every single minute of every single day. They don't need a national stage for their love. Families and loved ones need to do what works for them.*"

My mother has advocated for diabetes on the beach, standing at our beach blanket while my daughter and I played in the ocean. "*When I hear people say things, I'm not afraid to jump in and correct them, or strike up a conversa-tion,*" she said.

"Oh, you mean that time you had a long conversation on the beach with that lady who was talking about my insulin pump?"

"*Yes! She kept talking to her friend about how she was pretty sure you had a pump on and what she thought it did or didn't do. So I introduced myself as your mother and told her, 'Yes, that is an insulin pump.' And we talked for a few minutes about the pump, and the freedom it has afforded you. It could have been a really awkward conversation, but it was actually really nice. I'm always happy to educate on a person-to-person level ... especially if I hear someone talking about my kid's medical device while I'm standing right there next to them. Your whole family—your parents and siblings, and now your husband and your own daughter—are still waiting for type 1 diabetes to be cured. It's not going away. While we wait, we should find as much support as we can, and live well with this disease."*

Like me, George didn't know this kind of support was missing from his life until he stumbled into it. *"But once I found it, I realized that there are a lot of people who lived like I did, and still live like I did: feeling alone, isolated, and like no one understood them, in a diabetes sense. This hurt me because I didn't want anyone to ever feel like that— I knew how that felt, and it was an awful place to exist in. I want everyone to know there's a place here, a real community of people who live with diabetes, where they can feel understood."*

Being part of a community that understands how diabetes touches your life can provide the emotional support you may need to keep doing the necessary physical tasks.

The definition of our community is found in the people who are part of it. Each and every one of us—the bloggers, the lurkers, the medical professionals who care for us, the parents of kids with diabetes, the kids with diabetes who have grown up to become parents themselves, the lovers, boyfriends, girlfriends, spouses, friends of diabetics, the immediate family members and the ones who are slightly removed, the employers, the employees, the strangers who help us get juice when we can't help ourselves, the friends, Romans, and countrymen of the diabetics ARE the diabetes community. And everyone with diabetes, or touched by it, is able to raise awareness and make a difference, if that's their choice.

"All it takes is one other person to make you not feel alone," said Christel.

Chapter Fifteen

Taking Diabetes to College

I grew up in Rhode Island, a state known for Del's Lemonade and quahogs and the fact that it's the teeniest state in the United States. We're small, but proud. So going "far, far" away for college, to me, meant attending the University of Rhode Island (URI) ... a university that was, door-to-door, 30 minutes from the house I grew up in. (Stop laughing.)

When my acceptance letter came in from URI, with an academic scholarship attached to it, I was thrilled. This is exactly what I wanted—the chance to go away to college and earn a degree in English so that I could become a teacher. I wanted to live in the dorms and meet people and go to parties and live at the edges of "being an adult." And I wanted, and was ready for, diabetes to be solely mine.

My parents were thrilled that my grades were good enough to earn my admission to college, but there was a level of trepidation that they felt, different from when they sent my brother to college in Boston.

"When did you really have to let me go, diabetes-wise, Mom?"

"*Totally let you go? When you went college,*" my mom replied. "*But what made me feel safe was the fact that you were always making sure that you were safe, and that the people around you knew how to deal with diabetes-related emergencies. You weren't ever shy about telling people. Honestly, you never, ever didn't tell someone, when it came down to being close with them. School friends, roommates—even if you didn't like your roommate—you always made them aware of what was going on. You weren't ever ashamed of it, and you left little room for anything other than accepting it. Knowing your friends at school were well-informed made me feel safe.*" She laughed, ruefully. "*Safer, at least.*"

I remember talking with the Dean of Admissions about certain accommodations I was hoping to have in college. They agreed to put me in the freshman dorm, where the rooms were arranged into suites, ensuring access to a bathroom in the event that I decided to inject, etc., in the privacy of the bathroom. It was also decided that my diabetes supplies were to be kept in my dorm room in a lockable container, alleviating any fear of people stumbling across my syringes and lancets.

My mom and I purchased the biggest red tackle box we could find and a padlock to go with it from the local hardware store. It safely housed all of my diabetes supplies, from lancets to syringes. It was the oddest back-to-school shopping trip I had ever experienced.

In addition to this tackle box, I also had a Tupperware® container filled with low blood sugar reaction supplies. Fruit roll-ups, juice boxes, raisins, tubes of insta-glucose, peanut butter crackers ... it was a potluck of fast-acting, just-in-case carbs. And there were cake gel tubes to treat lows stashed everywhere. I had one in every purse, in my testing kit, the bedside table, the bathroom. I looked like I had a sneaky, little bakery fetish.

Aside from my cache of snacks, there were a few other tricks up my collegiate sleeve. Tucked inside my wallet, right beside my license, was a medical alert card that read, "My name is Kerri. I have type 1 diabetes. If I appear disoriented or intoxicated, please allow me to check my blood sugar as I may need sugar." I also had my trusty diabetes medical alert bracelet circling my wrist at all times. Emergency contact numbers were pasted to my computer tower.

All of my diabetes accoutrements were in order. All I needed to do was start disclosing my condition to my new roommate and my new friends. Without oversimplifying, the moments of disclosure were very direct, basic, and brief. Diabetes was something I was comfortable talking about, so it helped make it comfortable for them to hear. And within a few days, it became one of those "things in the background" that didn't become problematic except for a few instances.

But college, much like diabetes (or anything, for that matter) is different for everyone. There's no set rulebook that dictates how college should be tackled, or how diabetes should be handled. I spoke with three other college students (two having graduated and one currently in school) about how diabetes affected their college experience, and how they dealt with being out on their own for the first time.

Adam Brown, who graduated from the Wharton School of the University of Pennsylvania in 2011, found the college transition to be reasonably smooth. "*I was always very responsible and sort of took over my diabetes at a very young age, so the leap to college was not too dramatic for me,*" he said. "*I was diagnosed at 12 years old, and my mom always gave me plenty of autonomy. She was not a helicopter parent and never woke up at night to check my blood sugar, never asked me what my number was, and really let me handle the diabetes. I'm also the oldest of six kids, so my baseline level of responsibility was pretty high. Those factors combined to put me in complete control of my diabetes within about a year of being diagnosed. The big transition came when I went from injections to the pump—I don't think my mom had any idea how to work my insulin pump! Growing up that way prepared me well for having diabetes as a college student.*"

"*I was diagnosed at 14, a freshman in high school, and had the advantage of figuring out diabetes-related things by myself with my parents and family there to support me as needed,*" said Dana Lewis, a 2010 graduate from the

University of Alabama. *"As I moved into different stages of regular life—driving, going to college, and then moving across the country—I was lucky that diabetes itself wasn't an overwhelming challenge. I felt prepared and equipped to take care of diabetes. The biggest challenge for me was battling the label of what I thought being a person with diabetes was like, and the stigma attached to it.*

"My endocrinologist suggested a pump on the day I was diagnosed, and I was adamantly against the idea. A pump was a label and a huge screaming sign on my body that said I had diabetes, that I was not normal, and not like everyone else. I didn't want to tell many people after I was diagnosed, because it meant there was something 'wrong' with me. The biggest challenge was emotionally accepting the fact that I had diabetes and it was okay to be different, even if it was for a reason that I didn't self-select."

Savannah Johnson, diagnosed with type 1 at the age of two and currently attending Colorado College, realized right away that being self-sufficient bred ownership and responsibility for her. *"Being on my own actually did—and continues to do—innovative things for my diabetes in ways that the micromanagement inherent in being at home, under the care and responsibility of my parent, did not. Being at college means that my health, or lack thereof, is mine and I am responsible for successes and failures. I can't blame my parents' incessant questions or commentary or irritating nonverbal reactions to high blood sugars for anything; the questioning, commenting, and irritating nonverbal reactions, which are alarmingly similar, are mine to emit. And this was the first challenging yet refreshing realization I needed to ensure my health matched my health standards in college.*

College was not my first time being on my own. I had spent many summers prior to my freshman year working and living apart from my parents and family. But it wasn't until I arrived at college that I felt my diabetes was in my hands, and I would fight for every downgrade in A1C points because it was my battle."

For me, as a college student back in 2001, the access to unmonitored food and alcohol was a temptation. The much-discussed "freshman 15" didn't just threaten weight gain, but potentially a spike in my A1C percentages. (For the record, I never hit the teens in my A1Cs. I'm clarifying mostly because I know my mom is reading this. Hi, Mom.) Having grown up with type 1 diabetes, I had limited experience with drugs and alcohol, opting not to drink or smoke out of fear that I wouldn't be able to control my blood sugars. But being out of the house and out from under the watchful eye of my parents, I did try drinking alcohol. And it was always a carefully planned night.

"I know that you specifically chose the times when you would let loose and have a few more drinks. We would get super excited on those occasions that you were able to party with us," said my college housemate, Kate, one of the six other girls I lived with in college. *"That being said, I always*

thought you were a super responsible diabetic. It appeared to me that you knew your shit and did what you were supposed to do. At the time, I knew of another younger woman from home who also had diabetes and wasn't taking care of herself and wasn't able to get her numbers in check. I felt like you were super mature for your age and were able to take care of yourself and make good decisions in order to stay healthy. Your testing and injections were a normal part of our college life."

But even with a plan, things still weren't always properly controlled. *"There was the incident at the big party we had, where there was a mix up of your shots,"* recalls Kate, thinking back to the big party we had at our house our junior year of college.

At the time, my then-boyfriend had opted to remain sober and to help me check my blood sugar and take my nighttime shots (Lantus and Humalog, if needed). We had been dating for a long time and he was familiar with the process. But something ended up fumbling the works, and he accidentally injected me with a large dose of Humalog … instead of Lantus. The chaos that ensued was tremendous—unsure of what to do and too stupid to call for help, my boyfriend injected me with glucagon, since I'd been drinking. (We didn't realize, at the time, that alcohol impairs the liver to the point where glucagon is all but useless.) The glucagon shot made me throw up, which was a feeling exacerbated by the alcohol, so when the cops came by to break up the party, I was in a rough state. At the end of the night, my blood sugar was in the 200s and holding steady, and it had been hours since my last drink, but the lessons learned from a night of such irresponsibility and poor planning stick with me to this day.

"I'm sure if I wasn't impaired by alcohol and knew more of what happened I would have been more worried," Kate agreed. *"And now, looking back as a more mature adult, the situation as a whole is terrifying to me."*

Adam played it safer, and smarter, as a result of personal decisions. *"I decided that I wasn't going to drink alcohol. In addition to making diabetes control a bit more challenging, alcoholism runs in my family. At parties and social events, I'd always have to explain why I didn't drink. This wasn't a huge challenge, but it did sort of get old to explain my reasoning."*

But it wasn't just alcohol that proved challenging for Adam. He struggled with finding a doctor who fit his diabetes needs. *"Finding an adult endocrinologist was another challenge. I wasn't a big fan of the one I ended up going with. In fact, I would very infrequently make appointments, since I always felt healthy and never found them useful."*

Savannah, on the other hand, found herself completely immersed in college life and admitted to having trouble reminding herself that she had diabetes. *"I have also always been a very out-of-the-closet conversational type diabetic, so integrating diabetes into my social and romantic life was never a problem nor was ensuring my professors, coworkers, supervisors, friends, and partners were cool with my diabetes in the classroom, workplace, wilderness, and bedroom. Instead, I would say the most challenging aspect of collegiate diabetes was remembering that I do indeed have diabetes. And remembering that—like school, work, extracurricular, wilderness frolicking, and sexy time—collegiate diabetes takes time and deserves the time it takes."*

Then, after you adjust to the whole "diabetes is mine—almost exclusively!—to manage" aspect of living away at college, then there are the classes and academic workload that need to be managed. I found the chaotic triumvirate of working/classes/diabetes care to be an ultimate balancing act. So much emotional growth and physical chaos happening at the same time. How do you make sure your health or grades don't suffer?

For me, I also worked as a waitress throughout college, so my time was very full with school and work. But between my sophomore and junior year at college, my parents went through a very tumultuous divorce, throwing my world off-kilter for several years. Emotionally, I didn't handle this family dynamic change well, and my diabetes management suffered tremendously. People often ask if I had my highest A1C levels during college, and I have to say yes, but not for the reasons they assume. Dealing with so much college-related freedom, while also trying to wrap my brain around the fact that my home life was unrecognizable, was one of the hardest things I've gone through to date.

My last two years of college weren't like the first, and I was struggling to stay afloat more than anything else. I think the only reason my studies didn't suffer was because I threw myself into them to avoid focusing on my parents' split. But my diabetes care was all but ignored, and if it weren't for the Joslin Diabetes Clinic recommending that I spend a few visits with their clinical psychologist (the amazing Dr. Barbara Anderson), I may have taken even longer to get back on track.

Thankfully, not all college experiences include a family unhinging. Savannah chronicles her college experience by way of CGM mishaps. *"I'm pretty sure I can compartmentalize my college diabetic life into Dexcom-related debacles. The first would be when I moved to college as a freshman. I could have sworn I purposely put my sensor in a place I would be sure to not lose it, but alas, it was nowhere to be found post–move-in. The next would be after an unfortunate Camelbak water bottle leak into my Dexcom receiver on my second-ever backpacking trip. The third was a welcome-back-to-school night that I cannot tell you about, and the fourth was some time and place between Thailand, Laos, Vietnam, Cambodia, and the United States during which one or both of my sensors went AWOL. Through hours spent on the phone with insurance and many calls to campus safety to open up the mailroom on weekends, I realized that my key to the balancing act—especially during the transition periods of breaks, summer, class changes, abroad shenanigans etc.—was continuous glucose monitoring."*

For Adam, a few notable things kept his college experience on track. *"Always making time to exercise—I got into weightlifting my freshman year of college, as my roommate was a bodybuilder, and this profoundly changed my diabetes control. I also learned the importance of eating really, really well. I took some nutrition classes in college and completely changed how I ate. I had a realization that the fewer carbs that I eat, the less insulin I have to take. Not rocket science, but the key epiphany I had was that this reduces the potential for errors in insulin dosing. If successfully managing meals with diabetes is like firing a bow and arrow at a target, eating fewer carbs made the target much larger and easier to hit. And lastly, I always worked hard at my studies."*

One of the biggest challenges in transitioning to college can be the influx of adult freedom, which can be extra challenging for people with diabetes. Finding a strategy for being responsible at a time when perhaps peers aren't is crucial for staying on track health-wise.

"I tend to be pretty responsible, also known as 'boring' to some, and never felt the desire to experiment with illegal substances or completely go off the wagon, diabetes-wise," admitted Dana. *"There were definitely times where I would get burnt out and want to take the day—or week or month— off, and that's when I did the minimum to keep myself going but didn't think a lot about it. Then within a day or so, my brain would revive and figure out how to handle the stress*

again and let me return to normal management and decision-making processes related to my diabetes."

Adam found that developing good habits was his key to making the most of his college experience. *"Diabetes is such an invisible disease that you have to understand why good glucose control is important. I developed good habits in college—eating well, exercising, not drinking alcohol—that sunk in and have stayed with me over time. I thought of going to the gym like brushing my teeth or going to class—it was a non-negotiable and I never skipped out."*

"Luckily for me and my organs, I have really physio-emotional manifestations of hyper- and hypoglycemia," said Savannah, cutting right to the chase about what keeps her attention on diabetes while she's at college. *"Simply put, I hate being high and low. My body hates being high and low. I'm pretty sure my friends hate when I'm high and low. My mood, focus, homework quality, enthusiasm, motivation, and work ethic suffer when my blood sugars are not decent. Hence, I have never wanted to tell diabetes to go screw because I have never wanted to feel perpetually irritable, unfocused, academically unsuccessful, disinterested, unmotivated, and unproductive."*

Finding balance with diabetes at college can seem like one of those things that induces eyeball-rolls in many young people. "Sure, I'll just follow all these rules and be totally in-tune with my diabetes and not have a single blood sugar out of range. Oh, and I'll get straight As." I realize how over-simplified it can sound, at times. But college can be done—and done well—without putting your health or your future at risk—while having a good time, too.

"*It's important to think about the big picture,*" said Dana. "*Every day matters, but especially in the sense that it matters that you get up every day and try again. There will be bad days, but also awesome days where diabetes isn't the biggest thing on your mind. Take the good with the bad, and do everything you can to get up the next day and try again.*"

And both Dana and Adam feel strongly about diabetes not being a roadblock to having an awesome college experience—or an awesome life experience on the whole. "*When you really decide you want to run that marathon, you'll do it,*" said Dana. "*You'll figure out a way to rock a dorky belt with Gatorade, glucose tabs, pump, and your CGM for 26.2 miles and wrangle your BGs in the process. Diabetes definitely won't stop you from having an awesome career and a meaningful life. You'll meet someone who not only accepts you for you and your Diet Coke–drinking, Juicy-Juice-toting self, but also packs Skittles as backup for that umpteenth low and thinks your CGM is one of the coolest devices around. And your family will always be there for you, even if it's 2 A.M. and you need to wake someone up by phone to stay awake with you during a low. Thanks to them, you can do whatever you set your mind to—and you'll do it with or without diabetes.*"

"I did some cool and somewhat ambitious things in

college—studying abroad in Hong Kong and traveling all over southeast Asia, skydiving, backpacking in Europe for a month, a rock climbing trip in Mexico—so I don't have any regrets about missing out," offered Adam. *"Still, I think that's an important piece of advice for any college student, patient with diabetes, or a parent—don't let diabetes hold you back. Diabetes is not going away tomorrow, so why complain about it? It's a waste of time and energy and things that could be put to more fun-filled activities. You can travel anywhere in the world and do absolutely anything with diabetes. It's just a matter of being smart, being prepared, and planning ahead."*

Chapter Sixteen

Finding Balance and Moving Forward

It's a delicate balance, this one between "I'm sick" and "I'm fine."

"You have diabetes? You seem fine."

"I am fine."

On an average day, diabetes falls in the "annoying but tolerable" category. I check my blood sugar, wear any combination of continuous glucose monitoring device/insulin pump technology, do the insulin-to-carb math, eat well, exercise as often and as hard as I can ... the list is sizable and keeps me busy. For the most part, I don't see extreme hypoglycemia or excessive highs, and even though I see bits and pieces of diabetes in so many of my daily moments, it's not something that keeps me from pursuing the better parts of the day.

But on some days, diabetes falls into the "eff you and the effing islet you refused to ride in on" category. Those are the days when my infusion set cannula kinks up underneath my skin and sends my blood sugar cruising into the 400 mg/dL range. Or the days when a blood sugar of 38 mg/dL serves as a sweaty and panicked wake-up call at two in the morning. Or the days when I let my brain mull over the fact that I've had this disease far longer than I'll ever have anything else, and I fear the impact of these fluctuating blood sugars on my quality of life and longevity going forward.

It's a confusing shuffle, the one between feeling like diabetes profoundly affects my day-to-day health, both emotionally and physically, and the feeling that diabetes is just a blip on my daily radar.

"You seem fine."

I am fine. I think? I have a chronic illness—a disease—that compromises the function of my pancreas to the point where I need synthetic insulin daily, and even with dedicated management, I may see serious and debilitating complications in my lifetime. That's part of the dance—feeling and seeming fine and actually being fine, even though my body is dealing with something serious every moment of every day.

Is acknowledging that an invitation to feel bad for myself? No. But it's a reminder that even though I feel fine, and I mostly am "fine," there's a part of me that permanently needs tending to and ignoring it only leads to trouble. The low blood sugars and the high ones feel like they're ships passing by, but what they may be leaving in their wake scares me. I don't live with any difficult diabetes complications at the moment (though I do have macular edema and diabetic retinopathy, but these complications have not impacted my quality of life, to date), and my A1C is at a comfortable constant, so diabetes does feel quiet and well-behaved at the moment, even after 27 years. But I keep it on both the back burner and the front burner, knowing what this disease is capable of.

"I am fine."

Asserting that doesn't mean I want people to ignore the severity and pervasiveness of this disease. I don't want people who might be thinking about donating their time, energies, and finances to diabetes research, funding, and advocacy to be deterred by the fact that so often we look just fine. What those outside of this condition need to understand is that this perception of "fine" is all relative. One day you can be fine, and the next, life can be deeply and profoundly changed.

I've heard that fear is a pretty good motivator. Over the last almost-three decades with diabetes, I've heard the "fear tactic" from many medical professionals. Actual statements: "Make sure you test or your eyes will become diseased and you'll go blind." And, "If you don't take care of yourself, you'll lose a leg when you're older." And of course, "If you eat that, you'll end up with complications and then you'll have to live with that." (This is the diabetes equivalent of "Keep making that face and your face will get stuck that way." Eating does not cause complications; blood sugars consistently out of range do.)

Fear has never been a good motivator for me. It doesn't inspire me to try harder or to tap any source of inner strength. What fear does is make me want to ball up in the corner of a room and hide until the threat is gone or until the monster is shoved back underneath the bed. However, with diabetes, the threat isn't ever gone. It's always there, along for the ride even if it doesn't make any big moves. Being scared of diabetes doesn't help me manage diabetes. Fear gives diabetes too much power over me.

Coming up on 30 years with diabetes, I know what years with diabetes can do. I have sat in the endocrinologist's office far too many times to tune out the threat of "what might happen." And recently, I sat in their office and was handed a diagnosis of diabetic macular edema, which means that my eyes are starting to show the wear of so many years of type 1 diabetes, by way of protein deposits underneath the vision center of my eye.

Discussions about the elusive "what might happen" are often left in those quotation marks, as if that holds the threat captive. But let's be honest—after decades with type 1 diabetes, complications become part of the conversation. Retinopathy, kidney issues, depression ... the list is long and a good attitude, a determined mind, and even good control don't keep these issues entirely at bay. The best diabetes control isn't a guarantee, even though it is the best strategy. I've had my share of issues with my eyes. In the past, I've seen some cotton wool spots in my eyes. During the course of my pregnancy, retinopathy near the macula dictated a C-section delivery for my daughter. And now, a diagnosis of macular edema in my right eye.

This doesn't mean I've failed.

Finding balance and moving forward in a life with diabetes mean acknowledging these sorts of things, because it's real. It happens, and even though diabetes complications aren't necessarily guaranteed, they also aren't a mark of failure. I work hard to manage this disease. I will keep trying, even though I know there will be more radar blips and more moments that cause momentary tears but then renewed determination. There's so much personal responsibility, so many moments of "Well, you have the tools to manage this disease, so why aren't you hitting the mark?" Diabetes is unique, in that way, with complications often viewed as a result of the patient not working hard enough when in fact they are the result of diabetes.

Some people want to point fingers and to say, "Well, it won't be my kid," or "It won't be me." I can understand that. I didn't think it would be me. I hope it's not you. But it may be you, and in the event that it is, I want you to know that you aren't alone. Diabetes complications need to be talked about, because the guilt that comes with their diagnosis can be crippling, melting away the value of our efforts. It's easy to become overwhelmed when diabetes seems to be the leading cause of leading causes. For me, the diagnosis of macular edema made me want to wallow in self-pity for a while and hate diabetes, and I did that for a few days.

And then I moved on, because if I stay in that pool of guilt, I'll drown.

Fear is not the best motivator for me—hope is far more effective. I hope to be healthy for a long time. And it's hope that keeps me checking my blood sugar every morning, working with my doctor to best-manage diabetes, and monitoring this monster closely. I don't want images of amputation serving as motivation to grab my meter and check my blood sugar. I'd rather think about blowing out the candles at my seventy-fifth birthday party, a strong and healthy old woman.

Fear? No thanks. Show me people living well with diabetes, despite diabetes. Show me the people who are happy kids, or raising happy kids. I want to see the people who are working, traveling, exploring, and loving. Show me the people who are living with diabetes-related complications but still work to maintain their health and to live full lives. Show me people who don't view diabetes through a lens of shame and guilt. Show me that there is a life to be found after diagnosis.

Give me hope any day.

The concept of balance when tied to something like diabetes can sound laughable. Balancing a very needy disease within the context of a normal life can be done easily on some days and is impossible on others, making it maddeningly frustrating. On the days when diabetes is being needy, I feel weighted down by the prepositional phrase "with diabetes."

I'm a woman with diabetes. A mother with diabetes. A person with diabetes who had a crummy day with diabetes. I want to take one of those fancy knives they sell on late-night infomercials and slice "with diabetes" off the end of so many sentences. Balance, for me, comes from being Kerri. Not Kerri with diabetes, but simply Kerri.

Instead of viewing diabetes as my arch nemesis, I need to view it as my partner. (Or perhaps a business associate with whom I'm forced to work on a lifelong presentation?) Diabetes can't be changed, and even if I exercise violently every day and eat a raw food/paleo/ice cubes and biscuits diet for the rest of my life, my islet cells won't ever be reignited. Type 1 diabetes, barring a biological cure, is part of my life forever. Which is precisely why I can't hate it, either, because it's going to be around as long as I'm around.

Instead, I tolerate it.

This is reality. Anger doesn't do much for me in the long run. Frustrations ebb and flow, but in reality, those moments of burnout are fleeting. For me, it's about acceptance and healing. And realizing that it's okay to make mistakes.

Diabetes is a difficult journey. It is not a forgiving disease. It is something that must be monitored and maintained at all times, at all costs. It doesn't matter if you are shopping for your wedding dress, you must take into account where the insulin pump will hide. And happy birthday to you ... but if you have cake, you still need to check your blood sugar and take insulin to cover the cake. And if you want to have a baby, you can't just manage the pregnancy, but you must also manage diabetes.

Diabetes means living life on that seesaw. Some days you are way up high and other days have you almost in the dirt, both literally and figuratively. The constant efforts to keep the fluctuations of blood sugars to a minimum are just that—constant. The aim of diabetes management is to have that seesaw perfectly balanced, with a debate about the quality of life vs. quantity going on until the very end.

I can't let myself hate it, because it is a part of me. A part that I work so hard to maintain. And I will not allow one single part of me to root into a toxic panic that bores its way into my psyche. I am living with diabetes. And I will continue to live successfully for as long as I can.

How do I find balance? Honestly, I don't know. That's why the title of this book isn't *Balance: Found*. I search for it, though. I search high and low for the balance between feeling vexed by diabetes and feeling validated for all the work I do on a daily basis to take care of myself, and this disease. Sometimes I get angry that the reward for good behavior is the opportunity to try and behave all over again, and other times I'm grateful that I have the tools, technology, and support to manage diabetes.

Therein lies the balance, I suppose. Life with diabetes isn't about the diabetes itself, but about the life of which it's a part. There is a life to be found after diagnosis, and it's a damn good one. Being able to take a blood sugar and remove the blame and guilt from that result, focusing only on the actions needed to correct that number or duplicate it? That's balance. Viewing diabetes as something that doesn't define you, but instead simply serves to explain why glucose tabs live in your glove compartment and there is a pile of used test strips on the floor by your bedside table? That's balance. Being active and involved in a life that isn't ruled by insulin but is instead fueled by it? And realizing that diabetes isn't something we can perfectly control, but we can do our best to manage it?

That, to me, is balance.

There's a lot I can say about the diabetes community, and how far things have come in the last 27 years. How what was once a disease that left me feeling alone and obscure now comes with a welcome bag and a community of people who can lift your chin when it sinks to your chest. I thought about how many people I knew with diabetes on the day of my diagnosis (one) and how many I know today (far more than I can count).

I am grateful for all of these things.

Some years, on the anniversary of my diabetes diagnosis, I want to happily celebrate another year marked with diabetes. Sometimes I feel defiant, like I just poked diabetes in the chest and told it what's what. But some years, I want to keep to myself, feeling a little jumbled at the thought of so many years with this disease. And some years I'm a combination of all sorts of feelings, wanting my husband to give me a quiet hug and to avoid talking about it altogether.

I've wondered if maybe this day should come and go unnoticed, because an anniversary with diabetes doesn't change the diagnosis. Nothing changes ... right? Doesn't make my health any better or worse. It's just another box I can check, another year that I can say "Yes, I've been at this a long time." Maybe it's because I will wake up tomorrow and it will still be here, despite these promised cures. Maybe because I've moved into a brand new place countless times but still have boxes marked "diabetes supplies."

One time, as I was unpacking boxes after a move, I reached the bottom of a bin of clothes and found a used test strip. I couldn't even tell what kind of meter it went with, it was so old, and that made me so sad for some reason. I needed a hug. So I went into my daughter's room, who was five months old at the time. She was asleep in her crib, arms above her head, in her "sleep victory" position. Her breathing was even and steady, and she wrinkled her nose and rubbed her fist against her cheek as the floors yawned in response to my footsteps.

Diabetes may not define me, but my daughter does. My definition is found in those who love me, and in those whom I love.

I scooped her up without thinking and held her close. She cuddled close to me, resting her head against my neck and I stood there and felt ridiculous because I just wanted to cry, I was so proud of her. And so in love with her. And I realized that what changes, with each year marked, is everything.

Twenty-seven years with type 1 diabetes is a good chunk of time, but I'm not done yet. Diabetes is always there, but it's not me. It will never, ever be the core of me. Not if I have it for a 100 years. I remain in pursuit of balance, and always moving forward.

Acknowledgments

Thanks to the team at Spry Publishing for trusting me with this project and guiding me through the word-churning process.

Thank you to my brother and sister for continuing to support me, and thank you to my dad for raising me to refuse to back down (and to also pronounce my R's).

Endless thanks to my mother for coming to countless endocrinologist appointments with me, making that left-hand turn to the Joslin Clinic even though she was scared, forgiving me for lying about cupcakes, teaching me to respect myself enough to take care of this disease and trusting me to follow through, and now for being the best Grammie ever to my little Bird.

Thank you to those who have contributed to this book: my mother, my best friend, my siblings, Karen and Pete Graffeo, Briley Boisvert, Abby Bayer, Dr. Jill Weissberg-Benchell, Dr. Shara Bialo, Dr. Sean Oser, Dana Lewis, Adam Brown, Jacquie Wojick, Melissa Baland Lee, Lindsay Rhoades, Christel Aprigliano, George Simmons, Harry Thompson, Ginger Vieira, Scott Johnson, Kim Vlasnik, Katie Hathaway, Manny Hernandez, Savannah Johnson, Dayle Kern, Christopher "Sniffer" Snider, Ryan Noonan, Sara(aah) Nicastro, Christopher Angell, Blair Ryan, Jackie Singer, Laura Watson, Heidi Dennigan, Kate Mirabella, Lindsay

Swanson, and Karen Hoffman. You are all amazing friends, and I'm honored to have you as part of my life.

A big "no thank you" to my pancreas for hosting lazy cells, but a huge thank you to the diabetes community, who proves every day that there is a life to be had after diagnosis, and oh what a life it can be.

And lastly, thank you to my husband and my girl. I love you both beyond measure.